OBESITY
and its Management

Printed in Great Britain

OBESITY
and its Management

DENIS CRADDOCK

M.D., M.R.C.G.P., D.R.C.O.G.

General Practitioner, South Croydon

Foreword by
JOHN H. HUNT

M.A., D.M., F.R.C.P., F.R.C.S.

President of the
Royal College of General Practitioners

E & S LIVINGSTONE LTD
EDINBURGH AND LONDON
1969

TO MY WIFE
*who helped me with
much of the basic research
and encouraged me to
write this book*

Foreword

THIS volume should be welcomed by general practitioners and by hospital physicians as the first comprehensive monograph on obesity to be published in Britain or America for twelve years. The author, a well-known family doctor, bases his opinions on the results of his own follow-up of overweight patients over a long period; he compares fat patients with normal controls and he discusses a large series of weight recordings during normal pregnancy. For some of this work he was awarded, in 1968, the Hawthorne Clinical Prize of the British Medical Association.

After pointing out the size of this problem and its importance to family medicine, he discusses fully the complications and hazards of obesity, and its treatment by diet, drugs and exercise, each of which is given a separate chapter. Other parts of the book cover the aetiology and physiological aspects of obesity and its classification into clinical types. Long-term prognosis with and without treatment is examined carefully. Special interest is shown in decompensated and intractable gain in weight, and in weight control in childhood, pregnancy and in diabetes.

The Appendices should be useful for reference to many practising doctors. The first covers desirable weights (in pounds and in kilograms) for different age groups of men and women. The second lists the calorie values of common foods—something which many patients want to know but which their doctors may not always have easily to hand.

Dr Denis Craddock is to be congratulated on writing such a valuable book from general practice.

1969.   JOHN H. HUNT

Preface

SO far as I am aware this is the first time a general practitioner has written a monograph on obesity in the English language, and yet it appears to me that the physician in general practice has two advantages over the physician practising mainly in hospital, when surveying the treatment of obesity. Directly or indirectly the general practitioner sees almost every case of obesity in the community, while the hospital physician sees merely patients who are obese in addition to other medical conditions for which he is asked to give an opinion, or if especially interested in obesity he sees a small proportion of the severe or resistant cases from the catchment area of his hospital or hospitals. The general practitioner also sees his women patients during each of their pregnancies and has the opportunity, which is denied to the hospital physician, of influencing the eating habits of their families. Because of my position as a family doctor I have been able to survey all my treated obese patients over periods of up to ten years, and I have compared a consecutive group of 78, followed up for at least five years, with a control group. I have also recorded the weight gains in 100 consecutive ante-natal patients whom I have seen over long enough intervals to obtain adequate records, and have drawn conclusions as to the results of the dietary advice I gave to 60 of them.

Books on obesity can be divided into two main groups—those for the medical reader, and those for the lay reader. Books for the medical reader have in the main confined themselves to purely clinical aspects, whilst those for the lay reader have included considerable dietetic and nutritional advice. My aim in this book is to produce a comprehensive text book on obesity and, in addition to full clinical coverage, I have included calorie tables and various types of diet. I hope that physicians both in hospital and outside will find within its covers all they need to know for the practical management of their obese patients.

I wish to thank all those who helped me in the preparation of this book. Dr W. J. H. Lord of Alford, Norfolk, provided valuable constructive criticism of the thesis on which the book is based, and gave me ready access to his extensive bibliography on the subject. Mr D. Miller, Miss P. Mumford and Mr M. Stocks of the Department of Nutrition, Queen Elizabeth's College, London, gave detailed advice and constructive criticism on Chapters 5 and 8, and Dr D. A. Pike of King's College Hospital, London, advised concerning Chapter 16. Reg Finbow has kindly drawn the illustrations.

Others who assisted me in various ways were my partner Dr B. Barnes and my secretarial and office staff, Dr W. G. Christakis of New York, Professor C. A. Clarke of Liverpool, Dr C. Floyd and Miss J. Otway of Croydon, Mr J. C. Miller of Mayday Hospital, Croydon, Dr G. L. S. Pawan of The Middlesex Hospital, London, Dr W. G. Shipman of Chicago, Dr J. T. Silverstone of St. Bartholomew's Hospital, London, Dr A. J. Robertson of Liverpool and Professor J. Yudkin of Queen Elizabeth's College, London.

1969.   DENIS CRADDOCK

Contents

CHAPTER 1

The Size of the Problem

WHILE millions of human beings in the eastern hemisphere die from inadequate food intake, millions of their western counterparts eat too much, exercise too little and risk an earlier death than they need because of the ills produced directly or indirectly by obesity.

Before discussing the incidence of obesity in this country it is essential to make some definitions. Firstly, what do we mean by ' weight ' and secondly what do we regard as ' normal weight '?

What is body weight?

Physiologically the body weight is constantly changing, as intake of food and drink during the day is balanced approximately by loss of urine, faeces and of ' insensible perspiration ' at the rate of 30-60 g. (1-2 oz.) per hour. Under experimental conditions ' standard ' weight observations should exclude variables as far as possible, i.e. they should take place at a fixed time, preferably early morning, after urination and before food. In hospital practice weighing is usually carried out at a fixed time in a minimum of clothing, but in general practice, although the time can be arranged, routine undressing for obese patients is usually impracticable and the same type of clothing is usually specified for each weighing; normal indoor clothing for the time of the year is usual. Patients are not normally asked whether urine or faeces have been passed recently. As variables have not been ruled out, weight should always be thought of as ± 500 g. (1 lb.). Daily swings of water balance to that amount are to be expected and 1·4 kg. (3 lb.) variations are not abnormal (Strang, 1964). Over a period of years these variables cancel out and are unimportant.

1

What is normal weight?

Many of the older weight tables have been based on average weights for certain ages and have shown an increase in weight for each decade, whereas in fact the healthy non-obese adult should not vary in weight from the age of 30 onwards and probably from the age of 25. This theory has been confirmed by Slome *et al.* (1960) who have shown that Zulus living in rural areas and eating mainly cereals, fruit and milk maintain the same weight until the age of about 60 when the weight begins to decline.

In urban society, food intake does not usually diminish with increasing age, but physical activity lessens and weight is added. The Metropolitan Life Insurance Company of New York published a series of tables in 1959 giving the desirable weights for men and women over the age of 25 of small, medium and large frames (Appendix I) and these have now become generally accepted as the best yardstick for normal or desirable weights.

There is as yet no simple method for measuring an individual's frame to decide whether it is small, medium or large. Anthropologists take the bi-acromial diameter and the bi-iliac diameter as indications of the laterality of the skeletal frame, but even these require calipers to judge accurately (Montague, 1960) and 17 measurements are required for accurate somatotyping (Sheldon, 1954). Clinical judgment must therefore suffice.

What is obesity?

Most authorities define *obesity* as occurring when a patient's weight is at least 10 per cent in excess of the normal or desirable weight, although some take 15 per cent as the figure.

Clinical obesity is shown by an excess of subcutaneous fat. Except for short-term research projects there is no need to measure the thickness of skin folds by instruments and the diagnosis can best be made by estimating the thickness of the subcutaneous fat by pinching a skinfold in the mid triceps area, or below the scapulæ, on the lower part of the chest wall, the abdomen, the buttocks or thighs. Seltzer & Mayer (1965) have demonstrated that the triceps skinfold thickness is the best single criterion of obesity. Where the weight is 10 per cent above the desirable weight as shown by the Metropolitan Life Insurance Tables, the clinical diagnosis of obesity is rarely in doubt. The experienced clinician will not be misled by the increase in weight due to œdema fluid or excessive muscular hypertrophy. *Excessive obesity* can be said to be present when the weight is 20 per cent above the desirable weight, but some take 30 per cent as the figure. The United States Society of Actuaries (Metropolitan Life Insurance Company, 1960), taking the statistics of 26 large Life Insurance Companies in the United States and Canada, found the frequency of overweight and underweight to be as shown in Table I.

TABLE I

Percentage Deviation from ' Best ' Weight

Age	Men				Women			
	Above average			Below average 10%	Above average			Below average 10%
	10%	+10-19%	20%+		10%	+10-19%	20%+	
20-29	31	19	12	13	23	11	12	22
30-39	53	28	25	6	41	16	25	13
40-49	60	28	32	4	59	19	40	6
50-59	63	29	34	4	67	21	46	4
60-69	57	28	29	5	68	23	45	4

THE INCIDENCE OF OBESITY IN GREAT BRITAIN

McMullen (1959), defining obesity as ' a condition in which the body contours are distorted by a diffuse accumulation of adipose tissue,' surveyed 200 male and 200 female adult patients between the ages of 20 and 69 during a consecutive period in his general practice and assessed 9 per cent of the men and 27 per cent of the women as obese (18 per cent overall); only three of them had asked for treatment. Hopkins (1965) estimated that 20 out of 115 consecutive patients (17·4 per cent) were obese. Only two of these complained of being overweight.

How accurate are these estimates? McMullen appraised his subjects by eye and did not remove indoor garments, he used a table of standard weights prepared in 1943 and about half his subjects were above and half were below standard weight. These tables of average weight include all obese subjects and do not give an indication of ' best ' weight, nor do they take into account differences of body build. Thus some of his patients whom he estimated to be obese were not in fact overweight by his tables, and some of his patients overweight by his tables were not clinically obese. Hopkins merely ' collected the notes of 115 consecutive patients ' and found that in his estimation ' obesity was of importance in 20 of them '. He used a formula for estimating the average weight which included the addition of 500 g. (1 lb.) for each two years over the age of 20, perpetuating the fallacy that weight should increase with age. It follows that in both these studies the true incidence of obesity is underestimated.

The incidence of obesity in women

Silverstone and Solomon (1965) found that 15 per cent (41) of 272 consecutive women between 20 and 60 who attended the surgery of one of them were at least 12·7 kg. (28 lb.) above the best weight, according to the Metropolitan Life Insurance Society Tables. Adjusting Silverstone and Solomon's figures to 10 per cent above ' best weight ' about 21 per cent of their women between 20 and 60 would be obese. Few women in their twenties are obese, so that the incidence in women over 30 in this series is likely to be about 25 per cent. The incidence in the country as a whole is likely to be higher still, as their patients were mainly in social classes II and III which have a lower incidence of obesity than social classes IV and V. This is discussed more fully on p. 20.

In more recent surveys Silverstone (1968) found that 102 (56 per cent) of a 77 per cent 1 in 5 sample of adult women in two London general practices were more than 15 per cent overweight, and Hendry (1968) found 34 out of 100 women subjected to diagnostic screening in his general practice to be more than 10 per cent overweight.

In a survey of obesity in the author's general practice (p. 118) 14 of the women in the original control series were already under treatment for obesity, and of the remaining 56, 20 were found to be at least 10 per cent overweight. Thus 34 out of 70 original controls selected randomly were overweight. These controls are not a true sample of the practice population as they are weighted towards the age groups where obesity is most prevalent (Table XIII), but it is nevertheless likely that somewhere between a third and a half of the women over 30 in the practice are overweight.

It is likely that up to one half of the women over 30 in Great Britain are at least 10 per cent overweight.

The incidence of obesity in men

In the U.S.A. the incidence of obesity in men is almost as high as in women (Table I) but in this country it is considerably lower than in women. The author treated 15 men and 79 women in three years. McMullen (1959) found 18 men obese and 54 women, and Hodgkin (1963) encountered 122 female cases in one year and only 7 males. These three series together include 40 males and 255 females, a proportion of about one male to six female. This proportion is confirmed by the morbidity statistics from 100 practices published by the General Register Office (1958) so that it is likely that less than 10 per cent of adult males are overweight. Nevertheless in certain groups of men obesity can constitute a major health problem. In business executives, for instance, the incidence is high. Pincherle & Wright (1967) found that 567 (28 per cent) of the first 2,000 company directors examined at the Institute of Directors Medical Centre were at least 10 per cent overweight, the proportion overweight being almost identical in each of the age-groups, under 40, 40-49, 50-59 and 60 and over.

References

GENERAL REGISTER OFFICE (1958). *Studies on Medical and Population Subjects No. 14. Morbidity statistics from General Practice.* London: H.M. Stationery Office.
HENDRY, D. W. W. (1968). Presymptomatic screening. *J. R. Coll. Gen. Practnrs,* **16**, 45.
HODGKIN, K. (1963). *Towards Earlier Diagnosis.* Edinburgh: Livingstone.
HOPKINS, P. (1965). Obesity in general practice. *Proc. R. Soc. Med.,* **58**, 197.

McMULLEN, J. J. (1959). Obesity and body weight in general practice. *Practitioner.* **182,** 222.
METROPOLITAN LIFE INSURANCE COMPANY (1960). *Statistical Bulletin No. 41.*
MONTAGUE, M. F. A. (1960). *An Introduction to Physical Anthropology,* 3rd ed. Springfield, Illinois: Thomas.
PINCHERLE, G. & WRIGHT, H. BERIC (1967). Screening in the early diagnosis and prevention of cardiovascular disease. *J. Coll. gen. Practnrs,* **13,** 280.
SELTZER, C. C. & MAYER, J. (1965). A criterion of obesity. *Postgrad. Med.* **38,** A101.
SHELDON, W. H. (1954). *An Atlas of Man.* New York: Harper.
SILVERSTONE, J. T. (1968). Psychosocial aspects of obesity. *Proc. R. Soc. Med.* **61,** 371.
SILVERSTONE, J. T. & SOLOMON, T. (1965). The long-term management of obesity in general practice. *Br. J. clin. Pract.* **19,** 305.
SLOME, C., GAMPEL, B., ABRAMSON, J. H. & SCOTCH, N. (1960). Weight, height and skin fold thickness of Zulu adults in Durban. *S. Afr. med. J.* **34,** 505.
STRANG, J. H. (1964). In *Diseases of Metabolism.* Ed. Duncan, G. G. Philadelphia: Saunders.

CHAPTER 2

The Complications and Hazards of Obesity

THE statistics of the New York Metropolitan Life Insurance Company give the best approximation to the risks to life of obesity and its various complications. They show that the general mortality in the United States of America among obese men and women increases with each 10 per cent above best weight until, at 30 per cent above, in the age groups 40-69, it averages 42 per cent over average for men, and 36 per cent over average for women.

INCREASED MORTALITY

The increased mortality is brought about mainly by the increased incidence of hypertension and coronary artery disease. The Framingham heart study (Kannel *et al.* 1967) showed a dramatic increase in sudden death among men more than 20 per cent overweight as compared with those of normal weight and a lesser degree of overweight, and the mortality was reduced in those previously obese individuals of both sexes who had managed to lose weight. Marks (1960) quotes six sources from Germany, India, Norway and U.S.A. to show that obesity is associated with an increased incidence of hypertension and in this country Pincherle & Wright (1967) of the Institute of Directors found a diastolic pressure of over 100 in 84 (15 per cent) of 567 overweight men and in only 70 (6 per cent) of 1,225 men of average weight. The extra load on the heart and lungs of moving a fat thorax and pushing the diaphragm down against fat in the abdomen may also bring about cardio-respiratory failure (Berlyne, 1958). A hypertensive tendency can be present as early as the second decade, as Christakis *et al.* (1968) showed that in New York school children aged 10 to 13, 19·7 per cent of 74 obese children had a diastolic pressure of 85 mm. or over, as against

7

only 9·2 per cent of 556 non-obese children. This suggests an association between the hereditary tendencies to obesity and hypertension.

The greatly increased incidence of diabetes in long standing obesity is another important factor (Chap. 16).

TABLE II

Cause of Death in Men and Women Rated for Overweight

New York Metropolitan Life Insurance Company (Marks, 1960)
Based on 50,000 individuals who paid higher premiums on account of overweight 1925/34.

Condition	Men Percentage Actual Mortality compared with expected	Women Percentage Actual Mortality compared with expected
Cardio-vascular and Renal disease	149	177
Diabetes	383	372
Cirrhosis of Liver	249	177
Appendicitis	223	195
Gall stones	206	284
Cancer	97	100
Leukæmia and Hodgkin's Disease	100	110
Pneumonia	102	129
Ulcers of Stomach and Duodenum	67	-
Suicide	78	73
Accidents	(111)	135

Gall stones occur more commonly due to high blood cholesterol in most obese subjects. Liver damage leading to cirrhosis is more marked in men than women owing to their greater average intake of alcohol and consequent dietary neglect. The increased risk from surgery is due to greater technical difficulty and the increased risk of anaesthesia consequent upon an impaired action of the diaphragm. This increased surgical risk helps to double the mortality from appendicitis and gall stones (Table II).

Slower physical reactions help to increase the risk to life from accidents.

Obesity of marked degree leads to an increase in the complications of pregnancy and a higher perinatal mortality (Chap. 14).

THE BENEFITS OF WEIGHT REDUCTION

Reduced mortality

Men and women who lost weight and became accepted at standard rates by insurance companies achieved mortality rates approximating to those of people of normal weight (Marks, 1960). Statistics, as is well known, can give wrong impressions, and now that it has been established that there are at least two major groupings of obese people of which in one there are likely to be metabolic abnormalities which make it difficult for them to lose weight, it is possible to conjecture that those who lose weight easily would not be liable to much increase in mortality due to their obesity. On the other hand those who have abnormal metabolic factors are likely to have a high mortality which may be due to their abnormal metabolism rather than to their obesity. The probable linkages between hereditary factors controlling obesity and hypertension, and obesity and diabetes are relevant. Also ' women are fatter than men, but they live longer ' (Bruch, 1957). In drawing general deductions from insurance companies statistics, it should also be remembered that the overweight policy holders are not necessarily representative of the whole obese population.

Reduced morbidity

In general practice the main presenting symptoms are dyspnoea, pain arising from arthritic weight bearing joints, and gastric symptoms due to hiatus hernia (p. 127). The two latter groups of symptoms are productive of much distress although they do not lead to an increased mortality, and weight reduction will often lead to complete relief of symptoms or a major degree of amelioration. Hodgkin (1963) showed that fractures and severe limb injuries are much more common in the obese than in controls matched for age and sex, as also are prolapse and cystocele.

Gross obesity leads to a lowered fertility rate due to an increase in amenorrhoea. Of a group of 60 young women with amenorrhoea 48 per cent were obese, but only 13 per cent of a control group of 201 (Rogers & Mitchell, 1952). Amenorrhoea often develops following a sudden gain in weight; 15 obese women with amenorrhoea lost weight and 13 of them commenced to menstruate at the same time. Of 17 who did not lose weight only two commenced to menstruate again (Mitchell & Rogers, 1953).

None of the above conditions is likely to have much effect on mortality, but many of them have a great effect on human happiness as well as leading to loss of working time and it is here that weight reduction can have undoubted and immediate beneficial effects.

REFERENCES

BERLYNE, G. M. (1958). The cardio-respiratory syndrome of extreme obesity. *Lancet*, **2**, 939.

BRUCH, H. (1957). *The Importance of Overweight*. New York: Norton.

CHRISTAKIS, G., MIRIAJANIAN, A., NARTH, L., KHURANA, H. S., COWELL, C., ARCHER, M., FRANK, O., ZIFFER, H., BAKER, H. & JAMES, G. (1968). A nutritional epidemiologic investigation of 642 New York City children. *Am. J. Clin. Nutr.* **21**, 107.

HODGKIN, K. (1963). *Towards Earlier Diagnosis*. Edinburgh: Livingstone.

KANNEL, W. B., LE BAUER, E. J., DAWBER, T. R. & McNAMARA, P. M. (1967). Relation of body weight to development of coronary heart disease. *Circulation*, **35**, 734.

MARKS, H. H. (1960). Influence of obesity on morbidity and mortality. *Bull. N.Y. Acad. Med.* **36**, 296.

MITCHELL, G. W. & ROGERS, J. (1953). The influence of weight reduction on amenorrhoea in obese women. *New Engl. J. Med.* **249**, 835.

PINCHERLE, G. & WRIGHT, H. BERIC (1967). Screening in the early diagnosis and prevention of cardiovascular disease. *J. Coll. gen. Practnrs*, **13**, 280.

ROGERS, J. & MITCHELL, G. W. (1952). The relation of obesity to menstrual disturbances. *New Engl. J. Med.* **247**, 53.

CHAPTER 3

The Classification and Clinical Types of Obesity

CLASSIFICATION (AFTER MAYER)

GENETIC
1. *Simple obesity.* A multiplicity of genes.
2. *Associated with rare hereditary diseases.*
   (a) *Laurence Moon-Biedl syndrome.* Obesity, mental retardation, retinitis pigmentosa, polydactyly, stunted growth and hypogenitalism.
   (b) *Von Gierke's disease.* (Glycogen storage). Liver greatly enlarged, ketonuria, obesity.
   (c) *Hyperostosis frontalis interna.* Obesity occurs in less than half the patients.

HYPOTHALAMIC. Glycosuria and pyrexia usually co-exist.
1. *Traumatic.* After frontal lobotomy.
2. *Inflammatory.* Post-encephalitic.
3. *Neoplastic.* Invasion by malignant tumours of the pituitary.

ENDOCRINE. All these syndromes are rare. Wilkins, a prominent endocrinologist quoted by Savage (1968), had only seen two cases of Frölich's syndrome in 20 years of consulting practice.
1. *Fröhlich's syndrome.* This is commonly thought of in obese boys in whom the penis appears small as it is hidden in supra-pubic fat, but Scott (1966) says ' the syndrome should not be considered unless there is good evidence of an intra-cranial lesion '. The symptoms start at the age of three to six years and consist of obesity, sexual infantilism and impairment of growth. The fat impotent dwarf may develop bitemporal hemianopia due to increase in size of the tumour and may also have diabetes insipidus from hypothalamic involvement.

11

2. *Cushing's syndrome* usually occurs in females in the third or fourth decade. More than 50 per cent of cases are due to a basophil or chromophobe adenoma of the pituitary, and the rest are due to benign adenomas or carcinomas of the adrenal cortex. Increased secretion of glucocorticoids produces the well known syndrome of ' moon-face ', ruddy complexion, obesity especially of the trunk, purple striae, hypertension, osteoporosis, diminished glucose tolerance and amenorrhoea.

3. *Gynandrism and gynism* in which males have a mixture of male and female characteristics, sub-normal genitalia and obesity of Cushingoid type.

4. *Male hypogonadism.* About half of all eunuchs are obese, although they are not necessarily much overweight, as their muscle mass is reduced.

5. *Hyperinsulinism* due to tumours of the islets of Langerhans. The obesity is partly due to direct action of insulin in the formation of fat.

6. *Thyroid deficiency.* Myxoedema is not in fact usually associated with true obesity, except by coincidence. Myxoedematous tissue is associated with fluid retention.

7. *Stein-Leventhal syndrome* occurs in young women with secondary amenorrhoea, sterility, bilateral polycystic ovaries and sometimes obesity.

ANOMALIES OF FAT DISTRIBUTION

Lipophilia. Many obese patients show marked differences from the normal in fat distribution. In 41 out of a series of 200 adult patients surveyed by Rony (1940), 22 showed the upper body type where fat was distributed mainly above the waist, 13 showed the mid-section (' breeches ' type) affecting the buttocks and lower abdomen and six showed the lower body type affecting the pelvis, thighs and legs. Extreme cases of the lower body type have progressively less fat in the upper segment, and are then known as progressive lipodystrophy.

Some patients have exaggerated fat deposits in localised regions, such as below the chin, the buttocks, the trochanteric region or the lower abdomen. These localised deposits can be removed by surgery without recurrence. These abnormalities of fat distribution are genetically determined and sex linked.

Lipomatosis. A few people suffer from multiple lipomatosis. In many cases the lipomata are diffuse, about 5 to 10 cm. (2 to 4 in.) in diameter and painful. The case then constitutes the syndrome of adiposis dolorosa or Dercum's disease. The lesions appear suddenly, are red and firm and become painful and nodular. There may be spontaneous pain or severe tenderness on pressure.

REFERENCES

MAYER, J. (1957). Some advances in the study of the physiological basis of obesity. *Metabolism*, **6,** 435.
RONY, H. R. (1940). *Obesity and Leanness.* Philadelphia: Lea and Febiger.
SAVAGE, D. C. L. (1968). The fat child and the thin child. *Practitioner,* **200,** 361.
SCOTT, SIR RONALD BODLEY (1966). *Price's Textbook of the Practice of Medicine.* 10th Ed. London: Oxford University Press.

CHAPTER 4

The Aetiology of Obesity

OBESITY is particularly a problem of the affluent society with its high intake of sweet tasting carbohydrates and the generally reduced amount of exercise. Both doctors and laymen alike have been puzzled for generations as to why some people eating the same amount of food and taking the same amount of exercise as others can yet remain obese while their fellows stay lean. It has been shown in Chapter 3 that pathological and gross hormonal abnormalities as the cause of obesity are rare. Genetic, environmental and social factors are dealt with in this chapter, while physiological and metabolic factors are discussed in Chapter 5 and psychological factors in Chapter 9. Figure 3 illustrates the aetiology of simple obesity in diagrammatic form and can be found on page 41.

GENETIC AND ENVIRONMENTAL FACTORS

There is certainly a familial tendency in obesity. Several series have shown a greater incidence of obesity in the mothers, fathers and siblings of obese people than in normal, though the author can trace no series, apart from his own, which has been compared with a controlled series matched for age and sex. See Table III.

There has been much controversy about the relative importance of genetic and environmental factors in obesity, and the foregoing results have been postulated as being due to children acquiring the eating habits of their parents, rather than to them having an inherited tendency to obesity. Several lines of thought discount this theory.

1. *Studies with identical twins.* These show that there is a high correlation for weight between groups of twins despite environmental differences. This appears to be conclusive

14

TABLE III

Family History of Obesity

Series	*Subjects*	*Obese*	*Obese Controls*	*Normal Controls*
Hospital				
Gurney 1936	Parents	50/61 (82%)		18/47 (38%)
Rony 1940	„	175/250 (69%)	(24% both)	
Bauer 1945 (quoted Mayer)	„	730/1000 (73%)		
Gelvin 1957	„	34/39 (87%)		
Mullins 1958	Mothers	52/101 (51%)		19/50 (38%)
	Fathers	38/101 (51%)		1/50 (2%)
	Sisters	43/101 (43%)		14/50 (28%)
	Brothers	35/101 (35%)		2/50 (4%)
General Practice				
Lord 1966	Parents	24/28 (86%)		
Present Series	„	49/78 (63%)	14/28 (50%)	18/50 (36%)
	Sibs. and Children	55/78 (70%)	16/28 (57%)	21/50 (42%)

evidence for a strong hereditary factor. Newman *et al.* (1937), quoted by Rony (1940) and Shields (1962), surveyed 19 pairs of identical twins who had been separated from early childhood and lived in different families, mainly in different towns. Fourteen of the pairs were close to each other in weight, one pair differed by 8·6 kg. (19 lb.) but were grossly obese, one weighing 94 kg. (207 lb.) and the other 102·6 kg. (226 lb.). Of the remaining four pairs three had gross environmental differences; one sister of the remaining pair had five pregnancies and grew heavier with each, while the other had only one pregnancy. Newman also showed that the average pair difference is 1·9 kg. (4·1 lb.) for identical (monozygotic) twins against 4·5 kg. (10 lb.) for fraternal (dizygotic) twins, and 4·7 kg. (10·4 lb.) for non-twin siblings; only 2 per cent of the identical twins differed by more than 5·4 kg. (12 lb.) in weight against 51·5 per cent of the fraternal twins and 53·5 per cent of the siblings.

Probably the most conclusive twin studies of all have been those of Sheilds (1962) who showed that monozygotic twins brought up apart were closer in body weight than dizygotic twins reared together, the mean difference in weight between the 41 monozygotic twins being 4·7 kg. (10·4 lb.) and between the dizygotic twins 7·9 kg. (17·3 lb.).

2. *Gross differences in weight occur in siblings brought up in the same environment.* Astwood (1962) quotes a family of eight children, four of whom were of normal proportions, while the other four, who were not consecutive in family position, suffered from gross obesity; the patient aged 24 years was 207·5 kg. (457 lb.), a brother aged 21 was 154·4 kg. (340 lb.), a brother of 12 was 172·5 kg. (380 lb.) and a brother of ten was 124·9 kg. (275 lb.).

3. *The weights of adopted children show no correlation with those of their adopting parents.* The weights of natural children, on the other hand, correlate well with those of their parents (Withers, 1964).

4. *Inheritance of regional fat distribution.* Rony (1940), who made a special study of this subject, found that in 12 out of 18 cases of obesity of mother and daughter, there was ' unmistakable resemblance in fat distribution '.

5. *There is a strong correlation between body build and obesity.* Robinson & Brucer (1940) found that only 3 per cent of slender built men and 5 per cent of slender built women were overweight, whereas 37 per cent of broadly built men and 67 per cent of broadly built women were overweight. Seltzer & Mayer (1964) found that the bony dimensions of 180 obese girls were significantly greater than those of non-obese controls. As body build is inherited so must the tendency to obesity be inherited.

6. *Some children who are obese from infancy show a markedly increased carbohydrate tolerance.* Ellis & Tallerman (1934) showed that the average percentage blood sugar after a loading dose of glucose was only 120 mg. compared with 140 mg. of the other obese children. This is in keeping with the raised fasting plasma insulin level in some obese patients (p. 39).

The tendency to be obese thus appears to be inherited and Davenport (1923), quoted by both Rony and Gurney showed that the inheritance follows Mendelian patterns with the factors for stout build being generally dominant over the factors that make for a lean build. The factors probably number three or four. Gurney (1936) gave the results of pairings between stout and non-stout parents as follows:

Parents	Stout Children		Non-stout Children
Stout x stout	65	(73%)	24
Stout x non-stout	70	(41%)	100
Non-stout x non-stout	16	(9%)	160

How do these genetic factors affect the individual?

The following factors appear to be of importance:

1. ENERGY OUTPUT. Obese individuals tend to move less quickly than the lean and to expend less energy in sitting, standing and walking (p. 33 & Chap. 8). In the author's own practice two sisters separated in age by two years and brought up in an identical environment display these opposite tendencies. One moves slowly and puts on weight easily like her mother, while the other is physically very active and remains slim like her father.

2. APPETITE AND EATING HABITS. There is a range of normal in appetite as in everything else and this must be mediated by hereditary factors. At one end of the range the

TABLE IV

Eating Habits Compared

Habit	Obese Patients 78	Obese Controls 28	All Obese 106	Normal Controls 50	All Controls 78
Eating between meals	21 (27%)	14 (50%)	35 (33%)	8 (16%)	22 (28%)
Prefer sweet food to savoury	27 (34%)	8 (29%)	35 (33%)	11 (22%)	19 (24%)

' appestat ' is set so that the appetite is voracious. As Astwood (1962) says, ' it seems to me that *hunger in the obese might be so ravaging and voracious that skinny physicians do not understand it* '. Mall (1947) showed that food dislikes were doubled in individuals with slender and fragile bodies (' leptosomes ') compared with broadly built ' pyknic ' subjects. In the series in the author's practice (p. 118) more of the 78 obese patients and 28 obese controls admitted to eating between meals and to preferring sweet foods to savoury, than did the normal controls (Table IV). These results are significant when the tendency of obese people to minimise their food intake is taken into account.

3. DEFECTIVE ENZYME PRODUCTION. This may be a factor in some cases (p. 35). There are certainly metabolic factors in some obese people (pp. 39-40).

APPETITE AND SATIETY

The appetite regulating centre has been shown in experimental animals to be bilateral and centred in the hypothalamus (Brobeck, 1946). It is often called the ' appestat '. Damage to the hypothalamus immediately creates a voracious appetite. In humans this finding was first reported in 1840 by Mohr whose patient was found to have a pituitary tumour. There are probably separate centres for hunger (medial) and satiety (lateral). The mechanism for weight control is remarkably efficient in most people living normal, active lives, as the intake of merely 1 per cent excess calories each day will lead to a weight increase of approximately 0·9 kg. (2 lb.) in a year and 25·4 kg. (4 stones) in 30 years. The reason why weight is normally kept within such narrow limits over the years is not fully understood, and it may be due generally to an efficient mechanism for burning excess fuel rather than to controlled food intake (p. 33).

THE CONTROL OF APPETITE

Gastric distension. This leads to satiety and a diminution of appetite in most individuals. An acaloric meal of methylcellulose and water was shown to relieve the feeling of hunger for one and a quarter hours by Quaade & Juhl (1962). Hodges & Krehl (1965) found that their subjects were more hungry when fed a high sugar diet than when given a diet of the same caloric value consisting of carbohydrate in the form of vegetables and cereals. The complex carbohydrates may relieve hunger for longer time by distending the stomach for longer. The overstretched stomachs of some obese patients require a larger volume of food than normal to produce satiety.

Fat in the duodenum is the most potent inhibitor of gastric emptying (Campbell et al. 1968) and fat is usually the most satisfying food.

Hunger contractions may be part of the mechanism for initiating feeding, as they cease as soon as food enters the stomach; they are not an essential part, however, and they are inhibited by fear.

Blood glucose level. As insulin produces hunger when injected it might be thought that the hunger is due to the resulting hypoglycaemia, but if this was so diabetics with a high blood sugar level would never feel hungry. Mayer (1953) postulated that hunger was due to a low level of ' effective glucose ' which was the difference between the level of sugar in arterial and venous blood, but Quaade & Juhl (1962) found that individuals were still hungry after intravenous glucose had been injected. These findings do not necessarily invalidate Mayer's theory, as the hunger centre could be affected by hypoglycaemia without the satiety centre being affected by hyperglycaemia.

Blood insulin level. Insulin certainly produces increased appetite in individuals in a poor nutritional state and the high fasting insulin levels in the ' prediabetic ' obese (p. 39) may help to account for their hunger. Glucagon which increases the effective glucose level, depresses food intake several hours after it is given intramuscularly and it may oppose insulin in this way (Penick & Hinkle, 1961).

Blood NEFA level. A higher level occurs in starvation and possibly causes hunger by means of stimulating the appetite centre in the hypothalamus, while a low level occurs after a meal and is associated with satiety.

Rising heat load. Brobeck (1948) has suggested that we eat to keep warm as a fall of blood temperature stimulates the appetite centre, and a rise stimulates the satiety centre. This rise occurs after a meal, but it would appear to be too late to be the important factor in deciding when to stop eating, although it may lead to the spacing of meals.

Gastro-intestinal secretion. This, leading to tissue dehydration and satiety, may be the mechanism by which chewing and swallowing may lead to satiety without food reaching the stomach.

In western civilisation some individuals never feel hungry and some obese individuals never feel full or satisfied (Hollifield *et al.*, 1964), mainly because *the cerebral cortex commonly over-rides the normal physiological mechanism for appetite control*. In gross obesity food intake was shown to bear no relation to the state of the stomach, but was closely correlated with the quality of the food and the social circumstances surrounding food intake (Schacter, 1968).

Refined sugar, which is not a natural food for man, may lead to an increased food intake by increasing appetite, as suggested by controlled experiments by Yudkin (1959) and confirmed by a mass of evidence assembled by Cleave & Campbell (1966).

THE LONG-TERM REGULATION OF FOOD INTAKE

This is mediated by unknown factors. Taggart (1962) lost weight during the week and made it up at weekends. She did not feel hungry during the week or consciously feel hungry at the week-ends, and did not in fact realise that she ate more at the week-ends until her results were analysed.

SOCIAL FACTORS IN OBESITY

Obesity is a product of plenty, but social factors play a big part in determining the relative incidence in differing groupings.

Social class. In the City of New York (mid-town Manhattan area) a few years ago only 5 per cent of upper class women were obese, compared with 30 per cent of lower class women (Goldblatt *et al.*, 1965). The trends in men were similar though less marked. That the social pressures were the determining factors rather than racial groupings is shown by the decreased incidence of obesity among those who moved upwards in the socio-economic status from the class in which they were born (12 per cent) compared with those who remained in the same social class (17 per cent) and those who moved downwards (22 per cent). Wealthier families can afford the more expensive food necessary for dieting, and a slim appearance by a wife may be considered an essential contribution to her husband's success in business or professional life. The incidence of obesity is so high in the lowest social grouping that it is acceptable, and sometimes even considered praiseworthy, for women to be matronly in figure. In this country the same trend is present, although less markedly, the incidence of obesity being appreciably less in social classes I and II than in classes IV and V.

Silverstone (1968) surveyed two London general practices and found the incidence of obesity in social groups IV and V to be about 50 per cent while in groups I to III it was only about 20 per cent.

Recent immigrants to the U.S.A. had a high incidence of obesity, partly due to low initial socio-economic status, and partly due to the memories of recent hunger sustained in their countries of origin. In countries where hunger is common, the social incidence is the reverse of that in affluent communities, and success in life for a man is often measured by the girth of his wife or wives. In India, for example, Gour & Gupta (1968) found that of 68 obese patients attending the University Clinic at Aligash, 60 were from the rich and middle classes, 8 from the lower classes and none from the poor and very poor classes. By the time families had been in the U.S.A. for four generations, the incidence of obesity in women was only 5 per cent.

National habits. America is an international melting pot and in the mid-town Manhattan survey of 1660 representative adults there were nine ethnic groups. Among these only 9 per cent of the females of British descent were obese, compared with 27 per cent of those of Italian origin. The Italians consumed a greater proportion of fat in their diet than average, and welcomed obesity as a protection against tuberculosis. The Czechs love food and keep many of their traditional customs including a great deal of visiting on Sundays when large quantities of food are consumed, and it is considered impolite to refuse second or even third helpings.

Eating habits. Social visiting, with the hostess tempting the guests with delicacies having a high sugar and fat content and the guests eating more than hunger dictates out of politeness, is a potential factor in initiating or maintaining obesity in many cultures.

Most people, in their daily living, eat at habitual times rather than when they are hungry.

The media of advertising encourages the consumption of fattening foods. Life is hard for the dieting television enthusiast who has to sit through many minutes of tempting fattening food commercials between acts of his favourite play or show.

Social pressures affecting women. This is truly ' a man's world ' inasmuch as women suffer much greater temptations to overeat than do men.

They are usually the ones who have the daily temptations involved in the preparation of food. The products of stove and oven must be sampled, the food remnants left by the children must not be wasted and a meal must often be eaten with the husband as well as with the children.

A mother's life is more subject to minor frustrations and the constant decisions and responsibilities involved in looking after children of all ages. The boredom of daily household chores and sometimes, in addition, the strain of full-time work before the babies arrive and again when all the children are of school age make these women cry out for relief, and for many, eating is one method of obtaining solace.

When there are no children in the family or when children have left home and perhaps live far away, it is usually the women who bear the brunt of the emotional strain.

The ties of the family bear more heavily on women as a rule, and they have less opportunity for exercise to help them to keep slim. It is more often the man who gets the game of golf and almost all active sports have more adult male participants than female.

Manliness and virility are commonly associated with leanness, or at least an absence of gross obesity. Femininity on the other hand is associated with roundness and plumpness in most cultures.

Above all, however, women are subject to the metabolic changes of pregnancy and, in addition, to the emotional upset arising in civilised society from a first pregnancy which usually occurs five to 10 years after the physiological time of 14 to 16 years of age.

REFERENCES

ASTWOOD, E. B. (1962). The heritage of corpulence. *Endocrinology*, **71**, 337.

BROBECK, J. R. (1946). Mechanism of the development of obesity in animals with hypothalamic lesions. *Physiol. Rev.* **26**, 541.

BROBECK, J. R. (1948). Food intake as a mechanism of temperature regulation. *Yale J. Biol. Med.* **20**, 545.

CAMPBELL, E. J. M., DICKINSON, C. J. & SLATER, J. D. H. (1968). *Clinical Physiology.* 3rd Ed. Oxford: Blackwell.

CLEAVE, T. L. & CAMPBELL, G. D. (1966). *Diabetes, Coronary Thrombosis and Saccharine Disease.* Bristol: Wright.

DAVENPORT, H. (1923). *Body-build and its Inheritance.* Washington, D.C.: Carnegie Institute of Washington.

ELLIS, R. W. B. & TALLERMAN, K. H. (1934). Obesity in childhood. *Lancet*, **2**, 615.

GELVIN, P. & McGAVACK, T. H. (1957). *Obesity.* New York: Hoeber.

GOLDBLATT, P. B., MOORE, M. E. & STUNKARD, A. J. (1965). Social factors in obesity. *J. Am. med. Ass.* **192**, 1039.

GOUR, K. N. & GUPTA, M. C. (1968). Social aspects of overweight and obesity. *J. Ass. Phys. India*, **16**, 257.

GURNEY, R. (1936). The hereditary factor in obesity. *Archs intern. Med.* **57**, 557.

HODGES, R. E. & KREHL, W. A. (1965). The role of carbohydrates in lipid metabolism. *Am. J. clin. Nutr.* **17**, 334.

HOLLIFIELD, E., OWEN, J. A. & LINDSAY, R. W. (1964). Effects of prolonged fasting on subsequent food intake in obese humans. *Sth. med. J., Nashville*, **57**, 1012.

LORD, W. J. H. (1966). Health education about obesity. *J. Coll. gen. Practnrs*, **11**, 285.

MALL, G. (1947). Quoted by American Academy of Paediatrics. Committee on Nutrition (1967). Obesity in childhood. *Paediatrics, Springfield*, **40**, 455.

MAYER, J. (1953). Genetic, traumatic and environmental factors in the aetiology of obesity. *Physio¹. Rev.* **33**, 472.

MULLINS, A. G. (1958). Medical supervision in treatment of obesity. *Lancet*, **1**, 747.

NEWMAN, H. H., FREEMAN, F. N. & HOLLZINGER, K. J. (1937). *Twins. A Study of Heredity and Environment.* Chicago: University of Chicago Press.

PENICK, S. B. & HINKLE, L. E. (1961). Depression of food intake in healthy subjects by Glucagon. *New Engl. J. Med.* **264**, 893.

QUAADE, F. & JUHL, O. (1962). On the 'glucostatic' theory of appetite regulation. *Am. J. med. Sci.* **243**, 438.

ROBINSON, S. C. & BRUCER, M. (1940). Hypertension, body build and obesity. *Am. J. med. Sci.* **199**, 819.

RONY, H. R. (1940). *Obesity and Leanness.* Philadelphia: Lea & Febiger.

SCHACTER, S. (1968). Obesity and eating. *Science, N.Y.*, **161**, 751.

SELTZER, C. C. & MAYER, J. (1964). Body build and obesity—who are the obese? *J. Am. med. Ass.* **189**, 677.

SELTZER, C. C. & MAYER, J. (1965). A simple criterion of obesity. *Postgrad. Med.* **38**, A101.

SHIELDS, J. (1962). Monozygotic twins brought up apart and brought up together. London: Oxford University Press.

SILVERSTONE, J. T. (1968). Psychosocial aspects of obesity. *Proc. R. Soc. Med.* **61**, 371.

TAGGART, J. V. (1962). Diet, activity and body weight. A study of variations in a woman. *Br. J. Nutr.* **16**, 223.

WITHERS, R. F. J. (1964). Problems in genetics of human obesity. *Eugen. Rev.* **56**, 81.

YUDKIN, J. (1959). The causes and cure of obesity. *Lancet*, **2**, 1135.

CHAPTER 5

Physiological Aspects of Obesity

THIS chapter consists of a brief summary of the known basic facts concerning physiology and metabolism with which the practising physician should be acquainted in order to understand recent advances in knowledge concerning metabolic processes in normal and obese persons.

For a more detailed account of normal physiological mechanisms one of the standard works, such as Wright's *Physiology* or *Clinical Physiology* by Campbell, Dickinson and Slater should be consulted.

FATS

Physiologists refer to all fatty substances as *lipids* and divide them into the following groups.

Triglycerides (neutral fats). These are fatty acids esterified with glycerol (triglyceride alcohol) which is formed from glucose. Fats in foodstuffs and the fatty deposits of animals consist of mixtures of triglycerides.

Fatty acids are also known as non-esterified fatty acids (NEFA) or free fatty acids (FFA). Saturated fatty acids are solid fats and common members of this group are:

palmitic acid   lauric acid
stearic acid   myristic acid
butyric acid

Unsaturated fatty acids are oils which can be hydrogenated (saturated with hydrogen) to become saturated. They include:

oleic acid
linoleic acid, found in vegetable oils
linolenic acid, found in linseed and other seed oils
arachidonic acid, found in fish and animals

In the body nearly half the fat is derived from oleic acid, about a quarter from palmitic acid and the rest is a mixture.

Phospholipids. Fatty acids esterified with phosphoglycerol form the most important group of phospholipids which form part of the structure of cell membranes and are connected with the transport of fat about the body.

The sterols. These, including cholesterol, are solid alcohols.

ADIPOSE TISSUE

The ' adipose organ ' is now known to be a large and very active organ normally amounting to 8 to 20 kg. (18 to 44 lb.) in a healthy adult. It usually contains about 80 to 85 per cent fat, the remainder being cell material and supporting tissue. The protein content is about 2 per cent and water 10 per cent. The proportion of fat only increases slightly when the amount of adipose tissue is increased.

The metabolic functions of adipose tissue are:
1. assimilation of carbohydrates and lipids for fat synthesis and storage, and
2. mobilisation of lipids as NEFA.

NORMAL METABOLISM OF FATS

After absorption, mediated by lipase, fats are transported in the lacteals to the right subclavian vein and via the systemic circulation to the liver in the form of chylomicrons which are triglycerides with a coating of phospholipids. In the liver the triglycerides are broken down to fatty acids, and triglycerides are resynthesised in the proportions specific to man. From the liver the fats pass in the blood in the form of secondary particles (similar to chylomicrons but smaller) and low-density lipo-proteins (synthesised in the liver, bound to albumen and containing cholesterol as well as triglycerides and phospholipids) to adipose tissue where they are stored as triglycerides. *Fat storage is mediated via alphaglycerophosphate derived from glucose which has penetrated the cell wall aided by insulin.* Fat deposition therefore requires both glucose and insulin.

Normal blood levels:

Neutral fat (triglycerides) Fatty acids (NEFA)	200 to 450 mg. per cent
Phospholipids (including lecithin)	150 to 250 mg. per cent
Cholesterol & Esters	150 to 250 mg. per cent

Blood levels of a substance do not tell us what is happening to the substance; an increased blood level can be due either to an increased production of the substance or to diminished utilisation; this explains to some extent the differing results of different observers in this field.

Blood cholesterol levels. These are increased by any fats containing a high proportion of saturated fatty acid; these include beef fat and butter. They are also increased by a high intake of sucrose, but not by starch from cereals (p. 36). Thyroid hormones and physical exercise lower the level of plasma lipids including cholesterol.

The serum NEFA level is lowered by a meal, by glucose and by insulin; these act by inhibiting fat mobilisation and by increased re-esterification. From adipose tissue, after having been hydrolysed to NEFA, fats are carried in the blood, bound to plasma albumen, to muscle where they are oxidised to CO_2 and H_2O to provide energy.

The NEFA in the blood averaging 5 per cent of the total blood fat have a high rate of turnover (25 to 30 per cent per minute) and they thus act as a quick source of fuel.

Fat mobilisation. This is mediated by (a) *adrenaline,* (b) *nor-adrenaline* (released at the termination of sympathetic nerve fibres) and (c) *growth hormone* from the anterior lobe of the pituitary. Growth hormone acts as rapidly as insulin and promotes a brisk rise in plasma NEFA by taking fat out of store. This brisk response normally induced by hypoglycaemia (Luft *et al.,* 1966) is dependent on the integrity of the hypothalamus (Strong, 1968) (d) *ACTH* (e) *Thyroxine and tri-iodothyronine.*

Emotional stimuli increase fat mobilisation via adrenaline and growth hormone. Anxiety leads to increased NEFA levels within 15 minutes, but hostility has no effect (Cleghorn *et al.,* 1967).

The NEFA level is raised by starvation (there is a higher level in obese than in normal subjects which might be due to a slower turnover), by exercise when fat is being mobilised rapidly, and by diabetes, but the rise due to starvation, exercise, adrenaline, nor-adrenaline and psychological stress in the obese may be less marked than in the normal (Lennon *et al.,* 1967) partly due to less growth hormone being released.

FACTORS REGULATING THE LEVEL OF
FATS IN THE BLOOD

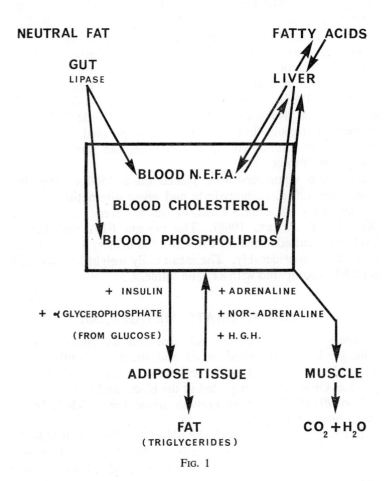

FIG. 1

Fat mobilising substance

This hormone, discovered by Chalmers, Kekwick & Pawan (1958) is produced when a carbohydrate deficiency exists (intake usually below 80 g. per day). In structure it resembles, but is not identical with corticotrophin (Kekwick, 1960). It releases fatty acids from fat and when injected into mice produces a rise in blood NEFA. It can be extracted from the urine and although it causes no diminution of appetite and no increase in oxygen uptake, i.e. there is no excess katabolism, energy is lost. The energy is lost via stools and urine in the form of complex organic carbon compounds (ketone bodies, citric acid, lactic acid, pyruvic acid). In mice the energy loss as expressed as a percentage of the intake is increased to 36 per cent compared with the normal 10 per cent on a diet containing about half the normal amount of calories (Kekwick & Pawan, 1967). The same effect occurs on a low calorie high fat diet (Kekwick & Pawan, 1966). Crude FMS was formerly antigenic but has now been purified and when injected into human volunteers produces the same effect as when used in mice.

Six obese volunteers were placed on a 1500 calorie diet containing 120 g. carbohydrate and given alternating courses of injections of either FMS or saline every second day (Kekwick & Pawan, 1968). The plasma FFA and ketone levels were raised while on FMS and the urinary ketone levels were raised considerably. The mean daily weight loss was 231 g. on FMS compared with 81 g. on saline.

CARBOHYDRATE METABOLISM

Sugars and starches are all absorbed as glucose, while cellulose is not absorbed at all and forms the bulk of undigested roughage. Insulin secretion is stimulated by the glucose. Glucose is transported in the blood and is

1. *oxidised directly by nervous tissue* for which it is the only source of energy;
2. *stored in the liver* with the aid of insulin, which aids the penetration of glucose into the cells, as animal starch (glycogen);
3. *stored in muscle* as glycogen or oxidised to produce energy;
4. *converted into fat* when in excess.

From the liver glycogen is converted back into glucose by adrenaline and glucagon, and the glucose is oxidised in the muscle to produce energy. If this takes place anaerobically, lactic acid is produced.

The human body is capable of a rapid rate of carbohydrate turnover; 2 or 3 g./minute can be oxidised and stored after a meal. **The carbohydrate handling capacity is lowered by infection or trauma, and increased by muscular activity or training, i.e. training in dealing with large carbohydrate loads (Beaudoin et al., 1953), as in a state of active obesity** (p. 35).

In starvation, when no carbohydrate is available, fat is changed in the liver to ketone bodies, βhydroxybutyric acid, aceto-acetic acid and acetone and these are used for energy, excess being eliminated in the urine (Kekwick, 1960).

In obesity, if a diet low in carbohydrate is taken, this elimination in the urine does not happen, due to adaptation, as the ketone bodies are normally used for energy (Kekwick & Pawan, 1957).

The regulation of blood glucose

Insulin facilitates the passage of glucose through the cell wall, glucose 6 phosphate is formed and adenosine triphosphate is converted to adenosine diphosphate. The blood glucose level falls.

Adrenaline produces a rise in blood glucose by releasing glucose from glycogen in liver.

Glucagon from the pancreas (a polypeptide) acts in the same way as adrenaline.

Cortisone slowly releases liver glycogen from protein and increases the blood sugar. (The use of protein for energy depletes the body protein store and this occurs on a very low carbohydrate diet, or if cortisone is taken as treatment.)

Caffein has recently been shown to increase the blood glucose level in maturity-onset diabetics (Jankelson *et al.*, 1967) and in normal volunteers (Cheraskin, 1967). It may therefore have a small part to play in the aetiology of diabetes.

Oestrogens may cause impairment of carbohydrate tolerance as shown by an increase in the blood glucose level during the premenstruum. Earlier reports to this effect were confirmed by Jarrett & Graver (1968). Oestrogens therefore are probably instrumental in hastening the onset of diabetes in the pre-diabetic woman during pregnancy (Pyke, 1956) and to a lesser extent on taking oral contraceptives (Wynn & Doar, 1966), especially mestranol (di Poala *et al.*, 1968).

FACTORS REGULATING THE LEVEL OF GLUCOSE IN THE BLOOD

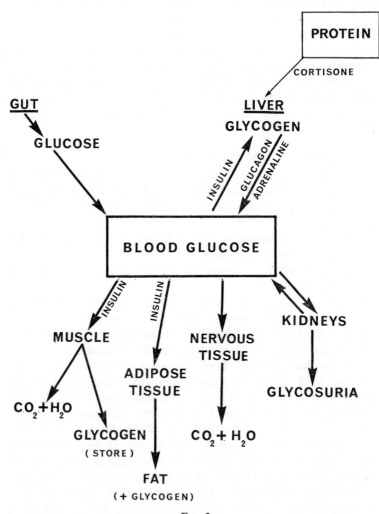

Fig. 2

PROTEIN METABOLISM

Proteins are absorbed from the gut as amino-acids and transported to the liver.

1. They are re-synthesised to proteins to replace protein breakdown (aided by insulin).

2. They are oxidised for energy, producing urea as a by-product.

3. They are converted to glycogen or fat.

The regulation of blood glucose and plasma free fatty acid

In the fasting state 70 per cent of the glucose output of the liver is used by the brain; it can only metabolise glucose. A low rate of insulin secretion and a low blood glucose concentration restrict the access of glucose to all other tissues.

Free fatty acids are an alternative source of energy.

When carbohydrate is absorbed from the gut the blood glucose rises. This stimulates increased insulin secretion and diminished release of growth hormone from the pituitary (and therefore diminished mobilisation of fat).

Liver glucose output is suppressed.

Glycogen and fat are synthesised.

Glucose is used instead of FFA as a source of energy by adipose tissue, muscle and liver. The serum FFA falls, and fat mobilisation is inhibited by insulin.

After absorption of carbohydrate has ceased, conditions begin to be reversed. The plasma insulin concentration declines, the secretion of growth hormone rises.

Fat is mobilised with the liberation of glycerol and FFA, which begins to be used for energy instead of glucose.

Glycogen synthesis ceases. The liver starts producing glucose again, the blood glucose and blood insulin levels then fall to the fasting norm.

Energy production

1. In the cell immediate energy is produced by the breakdown (hydrolysis) of esters, mainly adenosine triphosphate (ATP), an ester of phosphoric acid which is hydrolysed to adenosine, disphosphate (ADP).

Glucose + ATP → Glucose 6 Phosphate + ADP.

Some heat is already liberated, and this serves to maintain body temperature at the optimum level for metabolic processes.

2. The esters are then slowly reformed (e.g. ADP → ATP) by the oxidation of nutrients, mainly glucose, via pyruvate and acetyl coenzyme A.

This oxidation is mediated by five vitamins which form five coenzymes. Acetyl coenzyme A is oxidised in the citric acid cycle. It is formed in the liver and it is either

(a) oxidised to produce energy.

(b) hydrogenated in the presence of carbohydrate to produce fat.

(c) hydrolised in the absence of carbohydrate to produce free aceto-acetic acid (a ketone body).

There is a fine balance between the enzymes necessary for these three activities. If 15 per cent or more of the calories are in the form of carbohydrate (i.e. about 100 g. carbohydrate per day) as shown by the respiratory quotient of 0·75 or more, ketosis is prevented. The respiratory quotient is regarded as providing evidence of the source of the energy produced.

> Pure glucose produces an R.Q. of 1·0
> Pure protein produces an R.Q. of 0·80
> Pure fat produces an R.Q. of 0·7

THE MEASUREMENT OF METABOLIC RATES UNDER DIFFERING CONDITIONS

The basal metabolic rate utilised in experiments concerning obesity until 1950 or later is merely basic, as by definition the measurement of oxygen uptake is taken after resting and fasting for 12 hours. It is not very surprising therefore that the basal metabolic rate remains unaltered in cases of obesity as is confirmed by various studies between 1922 and 1950, nor is it increased by short term over-eating (Miller, Mumford & Stock, 1967).

There is no strict correlation however between the basal metabolic rate and the metabolic rate under more normal conditions. This was shown by McCance at Oxford after a series of careful experiments involving himself and his associates among a group of 22 men and 40 women (Boyens & McCance, 1957). In this small group the highest energy output for an individual member almost exactly doubled that of the lowest in each of the three positions of lying, sitting or standing. These findings have been confirmed by Durnin & Passmore (1967). *Many obese people with the same basal metabolic rate as normal individuals require less calories to maintain their weight as they utilise less energy when sitting, standing or walking.* The genetic characteristic of a tendency to move slowly is pertinent here (p. 17).

These findings also serve to confirm those of Widdowson (1947) who showed that for any given weight, age or sex it is possible to find individuals who customarily eat twice as much as others. Although the *basal* metabolic rate of obese people as a group does not differ therefore from normal, some obese people eat only half the amount eaten by lean persons of the same weight. The influence of exercise (discussed in the next paragraph) must also be considered.

Metabolic changes due to exercise and over-feeding

Miller and his colleagues (1966; 1967) working in Yudkin's department in London have confirmed quite conclusively that *exercising after food can dispose of excess caloric intake in the form of heat by approximately doubling the thermic response to a meal.* We now have a rational explanation of the fact that some grow fat while others of the same original weight stay slim on the same caloric intake. Miller & Mumford prefer the phrase ' thermic effect ' or ' thermic response ' to the term ' specific dynamic action of foodstuffs ' which was used previously and was thought to apply especially to protein. In fact, in their experiments with over-feeding, more weight was gained on a high protein diet than on a low protein diet.

In 11 young adults who over-fed for three weeks the basal metabolic rate was not increased. However, the thermic effect of a 1,000 calorie meal was approximately doubled by exercising after eating, the response being greater and longer lasting. Oxygen consumption reached its peak about one hour after the meal and was directly related to the calorie intake. The exercise, which was relatively mild, consisted of 12 steps of 11 in. per minute for half an hour and the thermic effect measured one hour after the meal showed a 28 per cent increase over BMR while resting and a 56 per cent increase while exercising. A total of 16 young adults altogether were over-fed for periods of four to eight weeks on low protein diets and after an initial slight gain in weight, the weight had become stabilised during the fourth week. Durnin & Norgan (1966) have confirmed these results in two out of three thin men.

Passmore *et al.*, (1955) found the weight gain less than expected in three thin young men over-fed for up to 14 days only, while in two fat young women (1963) the weight gain was as expected. This was probably because **obese people have lost the capacity to burn up extra fuel in the same way as thin people do.** This basic fact surprisingly enough was known as long ago as 1921 when Rolly (quoted by Miller & Mumford, 1966) showed that the specific dynamic action of foodstuffs was reduced practically to zero after the development of obesity.

Fryer (1958) gave 12 male college students a 1,000 calorie liquid supplement last thing at night for eight weeks. Each spontaneously cut down his intake during the day by an average of 500 calories, but the late night extra feed gave them no opportunity of exercising in order to expend the remaining 500 calories, and they gained an average of 450 g. (1 lb.) a week during the over-feeding period. However they lost an average of 900 g. (2 lb.) during the two weeks immediately following. In this country Ashworth *et al.*, (1962) also gave supplements at night and found that the gain in weight was much less than expected.

Metabolic changes in response to cold

The metabolic rate does not increase in response to cold in obese persons to the same extent as the normal. Quaade (1963) showed that a thick layer of subcutaneous adipose tissue and an ischaemic skin have an insulating effect against cold.

During a standardised exposure to cold, 10 lean persons more than 15 per cent underweight showed a metabolic increase of 33 per cent, 18 normal persons averaged 11 per cent increase and 16 obese patients showed an average of 11 per cent. However, 12 obese patients who did not admit to a great food intake (passive obesity) showed an increase of 2·5 per cent and four obese patients with a great food intake averaged 37 per cent (similar to the lean group) i.e. a state of ' active ' obesity. In confirmation of Quaade's work, Lennon *et al.* (1967) showed that plasma FFA level rose less in obese persons on exposure to cold than in normal controls, and Wyndham *et al.* (1968) showed that the metabolic rate of a man of average weight rose when the temperature was lowered to below 20°F (– 6·6°C) whereas in a very fat man this only occurred below 10°F (– 12·2°C).

METABOLIC DIFFERENCES BETWEEN THE OBESE AND THE NORMAL

In the majority of patients most metabolic differences between obese and normal people are ones of degree only and are due to adaptation to an abnormal intake of food at some time. It has long been known, however, that some obese people have greater difficulty in losing weight than others. It is thought that they may have basically inherited metabolic defects and it is possible that these may lie in the field of enzyme deficiency. Galton (1966) showed that in obese patients fat cells have a reduced ability to oxidise glycerol phosphate, by demonstrating a lower activity of the enzyme alphaglycerophosphate dehydrogenase. The glycerol is therefore available for fat synthesis and storage. Galton & Bray (1967) found that in three cases of obesity associated with intra-cranial lesions the adipose tissue behaved more like normal tissue and they argue that this suggests a basic enzyme deficiency in simple obesity. This may be the mechanism whereby a thermal response to food is less in the obese than in the lean.

The concept of ' active ' and ' passive ' obesity

All obese patients must at some time have eaten in excess of their calorific requirements in order to have put on extra weight. In particular there has been an excessive intake of carbohydrate. In this phase of weight gain one can be in a state of ' active ' obesity. At the end of this phase the weight of most obese patients remains more or less stationary for a time, and it is in this period of ' passive ' obesity that they do in fact eat less than normal people and yet remain overweight.

SUMMARY OF THE GROSS DIFFERENCES IN METABOLISM BETWEEN THE OBESE AND THE LEAN

While the basal metabolic rate is the same in obese persons as in the lean, there are the following important differences in metabolism between them.

1. Most obese people utilise less energy than the lean when sitting, standing or walking. — Genetic predisposition plus adaptation to a larger body mass.

2. Most obese people indulge in less exercise than the average, and consequently their metabolic rate fails to rise as much after food as with lean people. — Genetic predisposition plus adaptation, plus occupational and social habits.

3. Most obese people in the state of passive obesity fail to respond to cold with an increased metabolic rate as do normal people. — Adaptation mediated by a thicker layer of subcutaneous fat and an ischæmic skin.

Most obese people therefore in the stage of passive obesity genuinely eat only about half the amount consumed by lean individuals of the same weight.

In addition to the above factors it has been shown in the last 10 years that there are many differences between obese and lean persons in the detailed metabolic processes affecting both carbohydrates and fats.

THE EFFECT ON METABOLISM OF ALTERATIONS IN THE RELATIVE PROPORTIONS OF DIETARY CONSTITUENTS

A high proportion of sucrose

A diet containing a high proportion of sucrose leads to an increase in serum lipids while the same caloric intake of complex carbohydrates causes a decrease.

Yudkin (1957) first pointed out the damaging effect of

sugar on health. Keys *et al.* (1960) showed that sugar raised the serum cholesterol level, Winitz *et al.* (1964) showed that sucrose caused a rise but glucose caused a fall, and Hodges & Krehl (1965) found that sucrose raised the serum cholesterol level while a diet containing as much as 44 per cent of its calories in the form of complex carbohydrates caused it to be lowered (see also page 18).

McGandy *et al.* (1966) produced results which appear to contradict these, as they found only about 5 per cent difference in the levels produced by sugar and by cereals, but only the *mean* values of blood lipids were taken during short periods on sugar and starch whereas the *change* in values during short periods is more important, as a modification in diets takes several days to produce its full effect on blood chemistry. McDonald & Braithwaite (1964) found in seven normal men that sucrose caused an increase in serum triglycerides which did not occur with maize starch, and Cohen *et al.* (1966) found that both triglycerides and cholesterol in the blood increased sharply with sucrose and were lowered by starch.

Cohen and his colleagues (1961; 1963) made an interesting comparison between the dietary habits of the Yemenite Jews in Yemen and those who lived in Israel. The former had a much lower incidence of diabetes and ischaemic heart disease associated with low serum cholesterol and serum βlipoprotein levels. They eat similar amounts of animal fat to the Israeli Yemenites and had a similar intake of carbohydrate, but 20 per cent of it was in the form of sucrose.

What is the mechanism which brings about these differing effects? Davidson & Passmore (1966) suggest that the type of carbohydrate consumed influences the bacterial flora of the intestines which play a part in the absorption of cholesterol. The rapid increase in blood glucose caused by the quick absorption of sucrose compared with the slow increase produced by the slow absorption of starch from cereals may be another reason for the difference in their effect on serum lipids.

Vegetable oils and animal fats

Vegetable oils lower plasma cholesterol levels while animal fats tend to raise them. This fact is well established, although the significance to health of lowering plasma cholesterol levels is not yet fully defined, nor is the significance regarding weight reduction.

A high proportion of fat

This leads to a greater amount of ' fat mobilising substance ' being produced than on an isocaloric diet with a high proportion of carbohydrates and therefore the rate of weight loss is greater (Kekwick & Pawan, 1956). See page 48.

FREQUENCY OF FEEDING AND ITS EFFECT ON METABOLISM

Large meals lead to increased lipogenesis so that ' gorging ' has an effect greater than is expected from the increased coloric intake alone. This effect is mediated by a higher blood glucose and a higher serum insulin and can lead to a real weight increase as distinct from the apparent increase due to fluid retention following a large carbohydrate intake. Cohn & Joseph (1959) placed two sets of growing rats on an identical food intake. The set fed two meals daily showed a striking increase in carcase fat compared with the litter rats which fed normally by frequent nibbling. Other workers in the United States and elsewhere, and Kekwick & Pawan (1966) in this country confirmed their results. These results were confirmed in four obese human subjects by Gwinup *et al.* (1963). Comparing feeding one meal a day with feeding 10 meals a day over 14 day periods, they found that one patient on once-daily feeding showed a frankly diabetic glucose tolerance curve, and the other three all showed higher blood glucose curves on one meal a day than on 10 meals a day.

Fabry *et al.* (1964) in Prague assessed the frequency of feeding in 379 men and found that those who fed five times daily or more, were more successful in losing weight than those who fed three times daily or less. Lord (1966) found the same tendency in his smaller series. Miller, Mumford & Stock (1968) showed in over-eating experiments that individuals fed twice daily put on weight as expected, while if they were fed three times daily, or 14 times daily, the gain in weight was much less.

ALTERATIONS IN CARBOHYDRATE METABOLISM IN OBESITY

1. The fasting plasma insulin level is raised. This is so in more than half of non-diabetic obese (obese normal) patients as well as in most obese diabetic patients (Kreisberg *et al.*, 1967). During active obesity carbohydrate intake is greatly increased, which leads by adaptation to a more efficient and rapid removal from the blood (Beaudoin *et al.*, 1953). Increased insulin is necessary for this and can lead eventually to insulin resistance and diabetes in the normal patient. The islets of Langerhans were hypertrophied in 13 out of 19 of Ogilvie's cases (1935). The adipose tissue of extremely obese persons shows a decreased sensitivity to insulin in vitro (Salans, 1968). This fact may be due to the larger size of the fat cell in obesity, as it returns to normal with weight loss.

2. Hypoglycæmia occurs in response to a glucose load. This hypoglycaemic response to glucose occurs as a consequence of the raised plasma insulin level and was found in five out of 50 obese children in 1934 (Ellis & Tallerman) and confirmed in adults by Godlowski (1946) and more recently by Karam *et al.* (1963). Increased appetite may lead to carbohydrate addiction (p. 103). In obese diabetics insulin resistance has already occurred, and there is less response. The increased insulin response is abolished by phenformin in obese non-diabetic subjects as well as in diabetics (Grodsky *et al.*, 1963). The phenformin appears to act by increasing the oxidation of glucose in muscle. Butterfield (1967) thinks that this may be mediated by facilitating the passage of insulin through cell membranes. Increased lactic acid is produced as a consequence and a fatal case of lactic acidosis has occurred following an overdose of phenformin (Proctor & Stowers, 1967).

3. There is a low rate of oxidation of glucose, palmitate and βhydroxybutyrate (Gordon *et al.*, 1963). This arises out of the fact that *glucose uptake by muscles is decreased in obese non-diabetic patients and markedly decreased in obese diabetics* (Butterfield, 1965; 1967). This causes a diversion of ingested carbohydrate to adipose tissue. Butterfield & Whichelow (1968) found that the glucose uptake of muscle was increased when obese patients lost weight, and that fenfluramine also caused an increased uptake in five out of six obese patients.

4. The carbohydrate handling capacity is overloaded. In persistent obesity a gradual deterioration in carbohydrate tolerance occurs over the years. Ogilvie (1934) showed that after 18 years all his 11 subjects showed diminished tolerance, and three of them became diabetic. *Obesity therefore exerts a diabetogenic effect* (Chap. 16).

ALTERATIONS IN FAT METABOLISM IN OBESITY

1. There is a raised fasting free fatty acid level. In most cases of obesity this is so; it is decreased by phenformin. Carbohydrate is stored as fat, and fat is burned for energy in preference to carbohydrate and protein, as shown by a lower respiratory quotient when a standard mixed meal is taken.

The free fatty acid level does not increase in response to adrenaline to the same extent as normal in perhaps one quarter of obese patients, owing to impaired fat mobilisation (Gordon *et al.*, 1962). The level does not fall so much after glucose intake. Kneebone (1965; 1968) found that he could divide obese children into two distinct groups, in only one of which the serum free fatty acid level rose after oral glucose. The level does not alter with fasting.

There is also a raised serum cholesterol in some cases.

2. On starving the obese there is no ketosis (Kekwick, Pawan & Chalmers, 1959). There is also a low respiratory quotient as fat is being burned up and oxidised completely. By adaptation fat requires less carbohydrate when it is burned. It may indeed be converted to carbohydrate if necessary (Pawan, 1959).

3. The growth hormone blood level is low in obesity (Hunter, *et al.*, 1966). This means that fat mobilisation is impaired. In six out of seven normal men the level increased three to four hours after a meal. In the markedly obese fasting and exercise have no effect (Roth *et al.*, 1963).

OTHER DIFFERENCES IN METABOLISM IN THE OBESE

1. *Adreno-cortical hyper-activity.* In some obese patients there is an increase in 17 hydroxycorticosteroids in the urine with normal or low plasma levels associated with increased

THE AETIOLOGY OF SIMPLE OBESITY

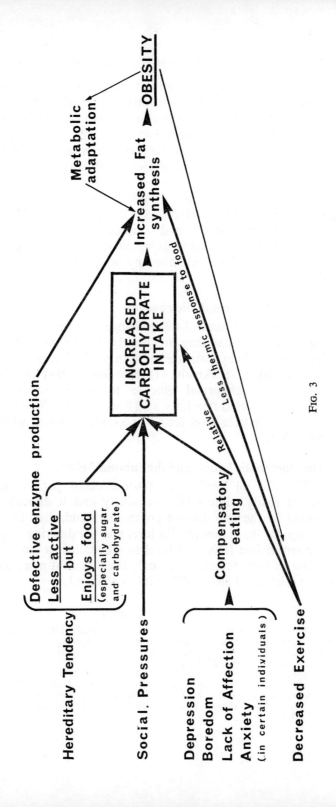

Fig. 3

cortisone production (Cohen, 1958). There is, however, no correlation with the degree of obesity (Schteingast *et al.*, 1963). 2. *A state of incipient iron deficiency* was found in adolescent boys and girls (Wenzel *et al.*, 1962). The Hb. was not significantly different, but the serum iron levels were 15 to 25 per cent lower than normal (Seltzer & Mayer, 1963). 3. *Renal blood flow and glomerular filtration are significantly reduced* and there is a high level of anti-diuretic hormone in the plasma (Bansi & Olsen, 1959). Fluid retention therefore occurs easily and is associated particularly with a high carbohydrate diet (Pilkington *et al.*, 1960); see page 48. This may be the mechanism by which hypertension is produced.

Reversibility of metabolic changes

The fact that most of these changes are reversible on losing weight proves that they are merely due to adaptation to an increased carbohydrate load and, in particular, to an increased sucrose load. Berkowitz (1964) found that out of 100 patients an abnormal glucose tolerance test was found in 58, an elevated free fatty acid level found in 70 and a raised serum cholesterol level found in 37; all improved with weight reduction.

The ' metabolic ' obese and the ' normal ' obese

The clinical findings that some obese patients can lose weight easily while others genuinely find it difficult, is confirmed by the two distinct groupings found, even in children, as regards the serum insulin level and the differing response of the serum free fatty acid level to adrenaline or glucose. Some obese patients therefore not only lay down fat more efficiently than others, but also mobilise it less efficiently.

REFERENCES

ASHWORTH, N., CREEDY, S. & HUNT, J. N. (1962). Effect of nightly food supplements on food intake in men. *Lancet*, **2**, 685.
BANSI, H. W. & OLSEN, J. M. (1959). Water retention in obesity. *Acta Endocr. Copenh.* **32**, 113.
BEAUDOIN, R., VAN ITALLIE, T. B. & MAYER, J. (1953). Carbohydrate metabolism in ' active ' and ' static ' human obesity. *J. clin. Nutr.* **1**, 91.
BENOIT, F. L., MARTIN, R. L. & WATTEN, R. H. (1965). Changes in body composition during weight reduction in obesity. *Ann. intern. Med.* **63**, 604.

BERKOWITZ, D. (1964). Metabolic changes associated with obesity before and after weight reduction. *J. Am. med. Ass.* **187**, 399.
BOYENS, J. & McCANCE, R. A. (1957). Individual variations in expenditure of energy. *Lancet*, **1**, 225.
BUTTERFIELD, W. J. H. (1965). Peripheral metabolism of glucose and free fatty acids during oral glucose tolerance test. *Metabolism*, **14**, 851.
BUTTERFIELD, W. J. H. (1967). The intravenous glucose tolerance test: peripheral disposal of the glucose load in controls and diabetics. *Metabolism*, **16**, 19.
BUTTERFIELD, W. J. H. & WHICHELOW, M. F. (1968). Fenfluramine and muscle glucose uptake in man. *Lancet*, **2**, 109.
CHALMERS, T. H., KEKWICK, A. & PAWAN, G. L. S. (1958). On the fat mobilising activity of human urine. *Lancet*, **1**, 866.
CHERASKIN, E. (1967). Effect of caffeine versus placebo supplementation on blood-glucose correlation. *Lancet*, **1**, 1299.
CLEGHORN, G. M., PETERFY, G. & PINTER, E. J. (1967). Studies in the autonomic. *Can. psychiat. Ass. J.* **12**, 539.
COHEN, A. M. (1963). Fats and carbohydrates as factors in atherosclerosis and diabetes in Yemenite Jews. *Am. Heart J.* **65**, 291.
COHEN, A. M., KAUFMAN, N. A., POZNANSKI, R., BLONDHEIM, S. H. & STEIN, T. (1966). Effect of starch and sucrose on carbohydrate-induced hyperlipaemia. *Br. med. J.* **1**, 339.
COHEN, A. M., NEWMANN, E. & MICHAELSON, I. C. (1961). Change of diet of Yemenite Jews in relation to diabetes and ischaemic heart disease. *Lancet*, **2**, 1399.
COHEN, H. (1958). 17-ketogenic steroids in obese children. *Br. med. J.* **1**, 686.
COHN, C. & JOSEPH, D. (1959). Changes in body composition attendant on forced feeding. *Am. J. Physiol.* **196**, 965.
DAVIDSON, Sir S. & PASSMORE, R. (1966). *Human Nutrition and Dietetics.* 3rd Ed. Edinburgh: Livingstone.
DI POALA, G., PUCHULU, F. & ROBIN, M. (1968). Oral contraceptives and carbohydrate metabolism. *Am. J. Obstet. Gynec.* **101**, 206.
DURNIN, J. V. G. A. & NORGAN, N. G. (1966). The effect of a period of overeating on the body composition of three thin men. *J. Physiol.* **188**, 26P.
DURNIN, J. V. G. A. & PASSMORE, R. (1967). *Energy, Work and Leisure.* p. 39. London: Heinemann.
ELLIS, R. W. B. & TALLERMANN, K. H. (1934). Obesity in childhood. *Lancet*, **2**, 615.
FABRY, P., FODOR, J., HEJE, Z., BRAUN, T. & ZVOLANKOVA, K. (1964). The frequency of meals: its relation to overweight, hypercholesterolaemia and decreased glucose tolerance. *Lancet*, **2**, 614.
FRYER, J. H. (1958). The effects of a late night caloric supplement upon body weight and food intake in man. *Am. J. clin. Nutr.* **6**, 354.
GALTON, D. J. (1966). An enzyme defect in a group of obese patients. *Br. med. J.* **2**, 1498.
GALTON, D. J. & BRAY, G. A. (1967). Metabolism of α-glycerol phosphate in human adipose tissue in obesity. *J. clin. Endocr. Metab.* **27**, 1573.
GODLOWSKI, E. (1946). Carbohydrate metabolism in obesity. *Edinb. med. J.* **53**, 574.
GORDON, E. S., GOLDBERG, E. M., BRANDABOR, J. J., GEE, J. B. L. & RANKIN, J. (1962). Abnormal energy metabolism in obesity. *Trans. Ass. Am. Physns*, **75**, 118.
GORDON, E. S., GOLDBERG, M. & CHOSY, G. J. (1963). A new concept in the treatment of obesity. *J. Am. med. Ass.* **156**, 50.
GRODSKY, G. M., KARAM, J. H., PAULATOS, F. C. & FORSHAM, P. (1963). Reduction by phenformin of excessive insulin levels after glucose loading in obese and diabetic subjects. *Metabolism*, **12**, 278.

GWINUP, G., BYRON, R. C., ROUSH, W., KRUGER, F. & HAMIRI, G. J. (1963). Effect of nibbling versus gorging on glucose tolerance. *Lancet*, **2**, 165.

HODGES, R. E. & KREHL, W. A. (1965). The role of carbohydrates in lipid metabolism. *Am. J. clin. Nutr.* **17**, 334.

HUNTER, W. M., FRIEND, J. A. & STRANG, J. A. (1966). The diurnal pattern of plasma growth hormone concentration in adults. *J. Endocr.* **34**, 131.

JANKELSON, O. M., BLASER, S. B., HOWARD, F. H. & MAYER, J. (1967). Effect of coffee on glucose tolerance and circulating insulin in men with maturity-onset diabetes. *Lancet*, **1**, 527.

JARRETT, R. J. & GRAVER, H. J. (1968). Changes in oral glucose tolerance during the menstrual cycle. *Br. med. J.* **1**, 528.

KARAM, J. H., GRODSKY, G. M. & FORSHAM, P. H. (1963). Excessive insulin response to glucose in obese subjects. *Diabetes*, **12**, 197.

KEKWICK, A. (1960). On adiposity. *Br. med. J.* **2**, 407.

KEKWICK, A. & PAWAN, G. L. S. (1956). Calorie intake in relation to body weight changes in the obese. *Lancet*, **2**, 155.

KEKWICK, A. & PAWAN, G. L. S. (1957). Metabolic studies in human obesity with isocaloric diets high in fat, protein or carbohydrate. *Metabolism*, **6**, 447.

KEKWICK, A. & PAWAN, G. L. S. (1966). The influence of feeding patterns on fat deposition in mice. *Metabolism*, **15**, 173.

KEKWICK, A. & PAWAN, G. L. S. (1967). Fat mobilising substance (FMS). *Metabolism*, **16**, 787.

KEKWICK, A. & PAWAN, G. L. S. (1968). Effect of fat metabolising substance in man. *Lancet*, **2**, 198.

KEKWICK, A., PAWAN, G. L. S. & CHALMERS, T. M. (1959). Resistance to ketosis in obese subjects. *Lancet*, **2**, 1157.

KEYS, A., ANDERSON, J. T. & GRUNDE, P. (1960). Diet type (fat constant) and blood lipids in man. *J. Nutr.* **70**, 257.

KNEEBONE, G. M. (1965). A biochemical, clinical and nutritional assessment of childhood obesity. *Aust. Paediat. J.* **1**, 120.

KNEEBONE, G. M. (1968). Drug therapy: an effective treatment of obesity in children. *Med. J. Aust.* **2**, 663.

KREISBERG, R. A., BOSHELL, B. R., DIPLOCIDOS, J. & RODDAM, R. F. (1967). Insulin secretion in obesity. *New Engl. J. Med.* **276**, 314.

LENNON, J. A., BRECH, W. J. & GORDON, E. S. (1967). Effect of a short period of cold exposure on plasma FFA level in lean and obese humans. *Metabolism*, **16**, 503.

LORD, W. J. H. (1966). Health education about obesity. *J. Coll. gen. Practnrs*, **11**, 285.

LUFT, R., CERASI, E., MADISON, L. M., VON EULER, U. S., DELLA CASA, L. & ROOVETE, A. (1966). Effect of a small decrease in blood glucose on plasma growth hormone and urinary excretion of acetylcholamines in man. *Lancet*, **2**, 254.

MACDONALD, I. & BRAITHWAITE, D. M. (1964). The influence of dietary carbohydrates on the lipid. *Clin. Sci.* **27**, 23.

MCGANDY, R. B., HEGSTED, D. M., MYERS, M. L. & STORE, F. J. (1966). Dietary carbohydrates and serum cholesterol levels in man. *Am. J. clin. Nutr.* **18**, 237.

MILLER, D. S. & MUMFORD, P. (1966). Obesity, physical activity and nutrition. *Proc. Nutr. Soc.* **25**, 100.

MILLER, D. S. & MUMFORD, P. (1967). Gluttony. I. An experimental study of overeating low or high protein diets. *Am. J. clin. Nutr.* **20**, 1212.

MILLER, D. S., MUMFORD, P. & STOCK, M. J. (1967). Gluttony. II. Thermogenesis in overeating man. *Am. J. clin. Nutr.* **20**, 1223.

OGILVIE, R. F. (1935). Sugar tolerance in obese subjects: a review of 65 cases. *Q. Jl. Med.* **28**, 345.

PASSMORE, R., MEIKLEJOHN, A. P., DEWAR, A. D. & THOW, R. K. (1955). Energy utilisation in overfed thin young men. *Br. J. Nutr.* **9**, 20.

PASSMORE, R., STRONG, J. A., SWINDELLS, Y. E. & EL DIN, N. (1963). The effect of overfeeding on two fat young women. *Br. J. Nutr.* **17**, 373.

PAWAN, G. L. S. (1959). The possible conversion of fat into carbohydrate in the obese human. *Biochem. J.* **72**, 20.

PAWAN, G. L. S. (1966). Effects of diet on carbon and energy loss in urine and faeces of man and the mouse. *Proc. Biochem. Soc.* **9**, 914.

PILKINGTON, T. R. E., GAINSBOROUGH, H., ROSENOER, V. M. & CAREY, M. (1960). Diet and weight reduction in the obese. *Lancet*, **1**, 856.

PROCTOR, D. W. & STOWERS, J. M. (1967). Fatal lactic acidosis after an overdose of phenformin. *Br. med. J.* **4**, 216.

PYKE, D. A. (1956). Parity and the incidence of diabetes. *Lancet*, **1**, 818.

QUAADE, F. (1963). Insulation in leanness and obesity. *Lancet*, **2**, 429.

ROLLY, F. (1921). *Dt. med. Wschr.* **47**, 887.

ROTH, J., GLICK, S. M., YALOW, R. S. & BERSON, S. A. (1964). Secretion of human growth hormone. Physiologic and experimental modification. *Metabolism*, **12**, 577.

SALANS, L. B. (1968). The role of adipose cell size and adipose tissue insulin sensitivity in the carbohydrate intolerance of human obesity. *J. clin. Invest.* **47**, 153.

SCHTEINGAST, D. E., GREGORMAN, R. T. & CONN, J. W. (1963). A comparison of the characteristics of increased adeno-cortical function in obesity and Cushing's syndrome. *Metabolism*, **12**, 485.

SELTZER, C. C. & MAYER, J. (1963). Serum iron and iron building capacity in adolescents. *Am. J. clin. Nutr.* **13**, 354.

SKIPPER, E. W., ORMEROD, T. P. & HASTE, A. R. (1968). Current therapeutics. 'Metformin.' *Practitioner*, **200**, 868.

STRONG, J. A. (1968). Human growth hormone. *Practitioner*, **200**, 502.

WENZEL, B., STULTS, H. B. & MAYER, J. (1962). Hypoferraemia in obese adolescents. *Lancet*, **2**, 327.

WIDDOWSON, E. M. (1947). A study of individual children's diets. *Spec. Rep. Ser. med. Res. Coun.* No. 257. London: H.M. Stationery Office.

WINITZ, M., GRAFF, J. & SEEDMAN, D. A. (1964). Effects of dietary carbohydrates on serum cholesterol levels. *Archs Biochem. Biophys.* **108**, 576.

WRIGHT, S. (1965). *Applied Physiology.* 11th Ed. London: Oxford University Press.

WYNDHAM, C. H., WILLIAMS, C. G. & LOOTS, H. (1968). Reactions to cold. *J. appl. Physiol.* **24**, 282.

WYNN, V. & DOAR, J. W. H. (1966). Some affects of oral contraceptives on carbohydrate metabolism. *Lancet*, **2**, 715.

YUDKIN, J. (1957). Diet and coronary thrombosis. Hypothesis and fact. *Lancet*, **2**, 155.

CHAPTER 6

The Treatment of Obesity by Diet

OBESE people have at some time eaten in excess of their energy requirements, and to remain overweight they must be continuing to eat in excess of their needs for their normal, or desirable, weight. The state of obesity has been described as the result of carbohydrate addiction (p. 103) and this observation helps to give an insight into the reasons why some obese patients are reticent about disclosing the amount they eat. Many feel frustrated knowing that they do not eat more than many slimmer friends. These sufferers have recently been shown to be correct (p. 36) and some consume only half the amount taken by other individuals of the same weight. Physicians in charge of metabolic units, however, are unanimous in their opinion that if a patient in hospital is not losing weight on a reducing diet, he is having food brought into him. In out-patients and general practice, similarly, if patients are not losing weight it is *usually* because they are unable to adhere to their diet. Many are too ashamed to admit to this in the same way that alcoholics and drug addicts will lie about the drug to which they are addicted.

FREE DIETS

Outside hospital a weighed diet containing a specific number of calories is not practicable for the general run of patients, and *Marriott's diet* (1949) impressed the author by the psychological value of its opening sentence ' eat as much as you like of . . . ' Marriott's was the first of the well known free diets in this country this century, but the first such type of diet to enjoy any measure of popular success was that published in 1864 by *William Banting* who had been given dietetic advice by William Harvey, an ear, nose and throat specialist whom he had consulted for deafness. Banting's high protein diet included some wine but almost completely excluded carbohydrates and fat meat. This diet was a more acceptable one 100 years ago as refined sugar, and products made from it, were not so much a part of civilised life as they are today, the consumption per capita having multiplied almost 10 times during the century (Cleave & Campbell, 1966). *The Prudent Diet* advised by the New York Bureau of Nutrition (Rinzler *et al.*, 1967) is based on similar principles. *Gordon's diet plan* (Gordon *et al.*, 1963) is similar, but emphasises the importance of eating six small protein meals daily. Roberts (1964) of Palm Beach, also feels that frequent non-carbohydrate meals form the best basis for the dietary treatment of obesity.

Free diets including fat

In America *Pennington* (1951) started from the known fact that Eskimos remained lean when their diet consisted mainly of fat meat, but became obese when traders introduced sugar and other carbohydrates into their diet. He helped to popularise a diet of 9 oz. of lean meat and 3 oz. of fat three times a day and advised in addition a 30-minute walk before breakfast. This type of diet suited many people in America, but it does not easily find favour in this country, and few of the author's patients have wanted to try it. That the diet still finds favour in the U.S.A. is shown by *Donaldson* (1963) who, after paying tribute to Pennington as a pioneer, advocates an almost identical dietary regime to his, adding six glasses of water between meals and potatoes or fruit daily.

Many doctors in this country have in the last 20 years produced diets based on similar principles to Marriott's, the most important modification being that by Professor *Yudkin* (1960) of Queen Elizabeth College, London, who advocates strict carbohydrate control and free intake of fat as well as protein. He assumes that on a long term basis people are more likely to keep to a palatable diet than one which requires stricter self control. As fat has a greater satiety value than carbohydrates (p. 19), the total calorie intake on a free diet like this is not likely to be great, and fat may have metabolic advantages over carbohydrate and protein (p. 27).

In six obese adults the total calorie intake was reduced by an average of 40 per cent over a two-week period as compared with two weeks on their normal diet and the fat intake was not significantly altered, being slightly increased in three and slightly reduced in three (Yudkin & Carey, 1960). Silverstone & Lockheed (1963) confirmed these results in seven obese diabetics using a diet containing only 50 g. of carbohydrate per day which was taken in the form of milk, Ryvita and fruit. Eating normal food there is an unavoidable minimum carbohydrate intake of about 20 to 40 g. daily.

Before the author had heard of Yudkin's work, he had already decided to modify Marriott's diet by adding 30 g. (1 oz.) of fat per day (p. 52).

In the U.S.A. Bloom & Clark (1964) found that four cases in whom there was no dietary restriction save for the removal of carbohydrate from the diet, all responded well.

Kemp (1966) has produced the best short term hospital results so far by treating his patients on similar lines to Yudkin, advising strict carbohydrate control, with a normal fat intake (p. 57). During 1956 to 1965 he treated 684 patients, who averaged six visits each and lost an average of 5·9 kg. (13 lb.); 63 patients were still under active treatment. Of the remaining 621 patients 239 (38 per cent) were successful in losing more than 60 per cent of the surplus weight, averaging 11·8 kg. (26 lb.) weight loss, 69 (11 per cent) failed, and 313 (50 per cent) defaulted and can be regarded as failures. (13, or 33 per cent, of the author's 39 patients with a medical reason for loss of weight had lost more than 60 per cent of their surplus weight after five years. This is considered more fully on page 127.)

The metabolic activity of a high fat diet. Kekwick & Pawan (1956) attempted to show that fats have a specific metabolic action, and they appeared to prove their point by showing that patients in their metabolic unit at Middlesex Hospital lost more weight on isocaloric diets high in fat and protein than on a carbohydrate diet. Moreover, Chalmers, Kekwick & Pawan (1958) showed that patients on 1,000 calorie diets excreted more fat-mobilising substance (p. 27) in the urine on a high fat than on a high carbohydrate intake. Pilkington (1960) at St. George's Hospital and Oleson & Quaade (1960) thought that their results might be due to alterations in fluid balance, and Werner (1955) had already found that high carbohydrate diets resulted in equivalent weight loss to high fat and high protein diets. Pilkington showed that patients on a high carbohydrate diet retain fluid, and on a high fat diet lose fluid, so that an apparent weight loss occurs on changing from a high carbohydrate to a high fat diet and an apparent weight increase occurs on going on to a high carbohydrate diet. This accounts for the fact that an obese patient who ' goes off the rails ' and eats a large carbohydrate meal puts on several pounds after one day or even one meal of over indulgence. He thus tends to lose heart unless he knows this fact about fluid retention.

Kekwick & Pawan (1964) restated their case for a metabolic difference occurring when isocaloric diets of different composition are fed. In mice given a high fat diet they found that more weight was lost than on a high carbohydrate diet of the same calorie content. In both cases the calorie content was about half of the normal intake of the mice. They proved that the weight loss consisted of fat by weighing the carcases after the feeding experiments. The difference they attribute to the effects of ' fat mobilising substance ' (p. 27).

Short term results of the free diet in general practice. *That the free diet is satisfactory for use in general practice is shown by the fact that almost every patient who takes his dieting seriously can lose weight for a month or two even if he has not the motivation to maintain dietary control for a longer period.*

In the author's main series, of the 76 patients who returned for early review as requested, 70 lost an appreciable amount of weight on a free diet: at least 1·8 kg. (4 lb.) in a month, 2·7 kg. (6 lb.) in two months or 4·5 kg. (10 lb.) altogether. Of the remainder four lost weight with the aid of drugs in addition to the diet.

The long-term effects of the free diet are discussed in Chapter 11.

Bulk as an aid to dieting

Many attempts have been made to popularise the introduction of indigestible material into diets as an aid to satisfying appetite, but they rarely work except for very short periods. One of the most popular of these is methyl cellulose which is made up in proprietary brands as either granules or tablets, and Duncan and his colleagues (1960) in a controlled trial, showed it to be ineffective compared with phenmetrazine and a dummy in 85 patients.

The following methyl cellulose tablets are on the market in Great Britain: Harley Discs, Kirby 10 Day, Limmits Pastilles, Pastils 808, Slenderettes, Slim-maid, Slimway, Slim Discs and Trihextin. The cost varies from 1d to 3d per tablet.

About 400 Consumers' Association members (1967) used one or other of these tablets, and among this group no more lost weight than among the 2,600 members who did not use them. Only about one in 17 found their hunger fully satisfied.

Special breads

Low carbohydrate (starch-reduced) bread which is also proportionately high in protein is advisable for most diets. The ' Cambridge formula loaf ' has recently been shown to give superior results to control bread over an 8-week period in 108 Cambridge patients (Howard & Anderson, 1968). One-third of them found the texture and taste unpalatable however.

Artificial sweeteners

Saccharine can be used *ad lib*. as it has no food value, and no side effects. Proprietary products based on saccharine include Biskoids, Energen, Hermesetas, Mini-Sax, Saxin and Sweetex. Most of them are considerably more expensive than saccharine.

Cyclamates produce softness of the stools and diarrhoea if taken in large doses, and it is unwise to replace more than 3·5 per cent of the sugar intake by them. The WHO Expert Committee has allocated to the cyclamates ' an acceptable daily intake ' of up to 50 mg. per kg. body weight, which is about 3·5 g. per day. Proprietary brands include Assugrin, Sweet'n'easy and Minnims. Up to 20 tablets can be taken daily.

Sorbital is an alcohol made commercially from glucose by hydrogenation. Most of it is absorbed slowly from the gut as glucose and metabolised. This slow absorption has little effect on the blood sugar level, so that it is useful in diabetes, but not in obesity.

DIET SHEETS

Details of the following diets are appended below.

Group A. Low carbohydrate, low or moderate fat diets

1. Marriott's Diet.
2. Author's modification of Marriott's Diet.
3. The Prudent Diet.
4. Gordon's Diet Plan.

Group B. Low carbohydrate, free fat diets

1. Donaldson's Anti-obesity Routine.
2. Yudkin's Low Carbohydrate Diet.
3. How to Lose Weight (Kemp).
4. Author's Present Diet Sheet.

Group C. Calorie controlled diets

1. 500 Calorie.
2. 1,000 and 1,100 Calorie.

MARRIOTT'S REDUCING DIET

1. Eat and drink as much as you like, or can get, of the following:

LEAN MEAT, including poultry, game, rabbit, hare, liver, kidney, heart, sweetbread, cooked in any way, but without the addition of flour, breadcrumbs or thick sauces.

FISH, boiled or steamed only—*not* fried. No thick sauce.

EGGS, boiled or poached only.

POTATOES, boiled, steamed or baked in skins. Not roast, fried or chips.

OTHER VEGETABLES, cooked in any way but without the addition of fat. Peas and beans should be omitted if weight loss is slow.

SALADS and tomatoes without oil or mayonnaise. Beetroots, radishes, watercress, parsley.

FRESH FRUIT of any kind including bananas; also fruit bottled without sugar. Not tinned or dried fruits (including dates, figs or raisins).

SOUR PICKLES—not sweet pickles or chutney.

SALT, pepper, mustard, vinegar, Worcester sauce (no other sauce).

SACCHARINE for sweetening. Water, soda-water and non-sweetened mineral water.

TEA AND COFFEE (milk only as allowed below), Bovril, Oxo or Marmite.

2. You may have milk (not condensed) up to half a pint daily.
3. You may have three very small pieces of bread daily. (Very small means 1 oz. or less), or six Energen rolls.
4. You may have *nothing else whatsoever.*

Note particularly that this means:

No BUTTER, margarine, fat or oil (except for cooking meat, not fish).

No SUGAR, jam, marmalade, honey, sweets, chocolate, cocoa.

No PUDDINGS, ices, dried or tinned fruits, nuts.

No BREAD (except as above) cake, biscuits, toast, cereals, oatmeal, Allbran, Ryvita, Vitawheat.

No BARLEY, rice, macaroni, spaghetti, semolina, sausage, cheese.

No COCKTAIL savouries, alcohol (beer, cider, wines or spirits).

Weigh yourself before you begin and once a week afterwards, on the same scales, in the same clothes and at the same time of day.

MARRIOTT'S DIET (MODIFIED BY CRADDOCK)

This is the diet used by the author in General Practice until 1967.

1. Eat and drink as much as you like of the following:

LEAN MEAT, including poultry and offal, cooked in any way but without the addition of thick sauce or stuffing.

FISH, boiled or steamed only.

EGGS, boiled or poached only.

SALADS (no mayonnaise).

VEGETABLES, cooked in any way, but without the addition of fat.

POTATOES, but not roast, fried or chips.

FRESH FRUIT, or fruit bottled without sugar but not dried or tinned fruit.

CONDIMENTS, sour pickles, thin soups, Worcestershire sauce.

THE TREATMENT OF OBESITY BY DIET 53

Tea, Coffee, Oxo, Bovril.

Saccharine for sweetening.

2. You may have:
    (a) *Half a pint of fresh milk daily.* (This includes all milk taken in tea, coffee, etc.)
    (b) *Three very small pieces of bread daily.* (Very small means 1 oz. or less), or six Energen rolls.
    (c) *1 oz. or less of butter or margarine daily.* (To be cut out if weight loss does not occur.)

3. You may have *nothing else whatever.*

    Note especially that this means:

    No butter, margarine, cooking fat or oil (except as above).

    No bread (except as above), Ryvita, biscuits (dry or sweet), cake, pastry, patent reducing breads (except as above).

    No sausages, cheese (except cottage), macaroni, spaghetti, rice, cereals.

    No sugar, syrup, chocolate, sweets, cocoa, jam.

    No alcoholic drinks.

    In other words, *nothing* containing sugar, fat or cereal in any form.

    Weigh yourself before you begin, and once a week (or once a fortnight) afterwards on the *same scales,* in the *same clothes,* and at the *same time of day.*

    On this diet you should lose between 5 and 15 lb. per month.

    Note 1. The weight can vary up to 2 or 3 lb. in the course of a day, usually being higher in the evening.
        2. A glass of beer or a short drink is equivalent in food value to 1 oz. of bread, and may be substituted for it.

THE PRUDENT DIET

This is used by the New York Anti-Coronary Club to lower serum cholesterol and also to reduce weight if the subject is obese.

This diet is essentially a low fat diet, with a relative decrease in saturated fatty acids.

MEAT—beef, mutton, pork: 4 meals/week.

POULTRY and veal: 4 or 5 meals/week.

FISH: 4 meals/week.

FAT: at least 1 oz. vegetable oil daily.

Margarine with high polyunsaturated fatty acid content. NO BUTTER.

MILK—skim milk only.

FRUIT ⎫
VEGETABLES ⎬ *ad lib.*

AVOID ice cream, hard cheeses, pastry.

For Weight Reduction Limit Intake to 1,600 Calories.

This diet averages 19 per cent protein, 48 per cent carbo-hydrate, 33 per cent fat. The fat comprises equal parts of saturated fatty acids, unsaturated fatty acids and poly-unsaturated fatty acids.

DIET PLAN (GORDON) (Author's Summary)

High protein	*Moderate fat*	*Low carbohydrate and salt*
100 g.	80 g.	50 g. (1,170 cal.)

Daily Food

At least six feedings daily each including protein must be taken including the following:

1. *One egg.*
2. *11 oz. lean meat*:

   6 oz. or more from Group A. Chicken, turkey, pork.

   5 oz. or less from Group B. Fish, lamb, veal, beef.

   In Group A. Instead of 1 oz. meat, one tablespoon of peanut butter, twice weekly.

   In Group B. 1 oz. cream style cottage cheese, or $\frac{1}{2}$ oz. cheddar, American or Swiss cheese, once a day, or one egg a day.
3. *Seven servings of fat.*

   One serving:

   1 teaspoon corn oil, cottonseed oil or safflower oil.

   * 2 teaspoons mayonnaise.

   * 1 tablespoon chopped walnuts or 4 half walnuts.

   1 teaspoon margarine.

         * not more than two helpings daily.

4. *Two cups skimmed milk.*
5. *Two servings fruit.*
>1 small orange, apple or fig (dried); 1 medium peach; $\frac{1}{2}$ small banana or grapefruit; 2 medium apricots, plums or prunes; 1 cup blackberries, raspberries, strawberries, rhubarb or melon; 10 large cherries; 12 large grapes; 2 dates; $\frac{1}{2}$ cup orange or grapefruit juice; 2 tablespoons raisins.
6. *Two to four cups vegetables. Group A.*
>Asparagus, cabbage or other greens, celery, chicory, cucumber, egg plant, lettuce, mushrooms, peppers, radishes, runner beans, tomatoes, mustard, cress.
7. *One half-slice bread.*
>or
>
>*One half-cup vegetables. Group B.*
>Beet, carrots, onions, peas, turnip, pumpkin.

Suggested Daily Meal Plan

BREAKFAST
>$\frac{1}{2}$ cup fruit juice; 1 egg; 1 oz. meat; 1 teaspoon margarine; $\frac{1}{2}$ slice bread; coffee or tea.

MID-MORNING
>1 cup skimmed milk; 1 oz. meat.

LUNCH
>3 oz. meat; vegetable A; 1 teaspoon margarine; 2 teaspoons corn oil; coffee or tea.

MID-AFTERNOON
>2 oz. meat; $\frac{1}{2}$ cup skimmed milk.

DINNER
>3 oz. meat; vegetable A; 1 teaspoon margarine; 2 teaspoons corn oil; 1 serving fruit; coffee or tea.

EVENING
>$\frac{1}{2}$ cup skimmed milk; 1 oz. meat.

DONALDSON'S ANTI-OBESITY ROUTINE
(Author's Summary)

1. Eat three times daily
>(a) 8 oz. of fresh fat meat without salt (to contain after cooking 2 oz. of fat, 6 oz. of lean).

(b) a hotel portion of ripe, raw fruit *or* a potato baked or boiled without salt.

(c) a half-cup of black coffee *or* a full cup of clear tea.

2. Drink six glasses of water between meals by 5 o'clock in the afternoon.
3. Walk for 30 minutes before breakfast each day.
4. Sleep for six to eight hours each night.

YUDKIN'S LOW CARBOHYDRATE DIET
(Author's Summary)

Each carbohydrate unit (C.U.) is the equivalent of 5 g. of carbohydrate (20 calories). See Appendix II for details.

1. Cut your carbohydrate allowance to 15 C.U's a day (300 calories) and if you are losing weight too slowly, to 10 or even less.
2. You should have foods from each of the basic four groups twice a day.
    Group 1. Milk and cheese.
    Group 2. Meat, fish, eggs.
    Group 3. Fruit, vegetables.
    Group 4. Butter, margarine.
    You should take half to one pint of milk daily.

Sample C.U. Diet

BREAKFAST
Half a grapefruit; egg and bacon; bread (one slice); butter; tea or coffee.

MID-MORNING
Tea or Coffee.

LUNCH
Stewed beef; brussel sprouts; starch reduced rolls (two); butter; fresh fruit salad with cream.

TEA
Tea and one sweet biscuit.

DINNER
Grilled fish; spinach; potato (one medium); starch reduced rolls; butter; cheese.

BED-TIME
Cocoa.

How to Lose Weight (Kemp)
(Author's Summary)

1. The principle of this diet is the avoidance of all starch and sugar but with an increased amount of meat and protein and a normal amount of fatty foods.
2. You must give up everything containing sugar or made of flour, instead of bread you must eat only starch reduced rolls or crisp bread. Saccharine can be used instead of sugar and diabetic preparations such as jams are allowed.
3. Plenty of all kinds of vegetables except potatoes are needed. As many salads and as much fruit as possible should be eaten.
4. You must eat more than your usual amounts of meat, fish, cheese, eggs, bacon, ham.
5. Butter, margarine and cooking fats need not be limited.
6. As far as drinks are concerned you should limit your milk to $\frac{1}{2}$ pint a day and avoid beer, stout or cider.
7. Increased activity, e.g. walking instead of taking a 'bus will help but strenuous exercise is not likely to be of much use.
8. Have three or four good meals a day of non-fattening foods. There is never any need to be hungry. Never try to live on a low calorie starvation diet. There is no need to limit salt or the amount of fluid you drink.
9. Weight reduction needs to be slow and steady. Once weight has been lost you must never go back to the old type of meals. Fat people cannot deal with ordinary amounts of sugar and starch without turning it into fat, so that it will be necessary to choose your food and watch your weight indefinitely.

Author's Present Diet Sheet

1. Eat and drink as much as you like of the following:
   Lean Meat, including poultry and offal.
   Fish.
   Eggs.
   Cheese.
   Salads.
   Vegetables.

FRESH FRUIT or fruit bottled without sugar, but not dried or tinned fruit.

BUTTER, margarine and cooking fat.

CONDIMENTS, sour pickles, thin soups, Worcestershire sauce.

TEA, coffee, Oxo, Bovril.

SACCHARINE for sweetening.

2. You may have:
   (a) ½ pint of fresh milk daily. (This includes all milk taken in tea, coffee, etc.).
   (b) Up to 3 oz. of reducing bread, or crisp bread, or six Energen rolls daily.
   (c) One or two small potatoes per helping.

3. You may have *nothing else whatever*.

   Note especially that this means:

   No bread (except as above), biscuits (dry or sweet), cake or pastry.

   No sausages, macaroni, spaghetti, rice, cereals, thick sauces.

   No sugar, syrup, chocolate, sweets, cocoa, honey, jam (except diabetic).

   No alcoholic drink.

   In Other Words Nothing Containing Sugar or Cereal in Any Form.

   Weigh yourself before you begin, and once a week or once a fortnight afterwards, on the *same scales,* in the *same clothes* and at the *same time of day.*

   You should eat three or four meals a day.

   On this diet, you should lose between 5 and 10 lb. per month.

NOTE:

1. The weight can vary up to 2 or 3 lb. in the course of a day, usually being higher in the evening.

2. A glass of beer or a short drink is equivalent in food value to 1 oz. of bread, and may be substituted for it. A drink is best taken with the evening meal.

The Importance of Exercise in Weight Reduction

A person weighing 10 stone who walks an extra three miles each day, or cycles for three-quarters of an hour daily, or swims or plays tennis for half an hour daily, will lose *at least* 3 lb. a month, as well as any weight lost by dieting.

Recent research has shown that more weight is lost by exercise if it is taken one to two hours after food, as some of the food is turned into heat instead of fat.

CALORIE CONTROLLED DIETS

Some patients can lose weight better by being given a more detailed diet, to which they endeavour to adhere. Even in hospital practice, however, there are a large number of defaulters from a sub-caloric diet: 239 out of 1,000 consecutive patients defaulted in the Edinburgh series of Seaton & Rose (1965). The following diets taken from Strang (1964) are examples of the amount of food which is contained in 500 and 1,000 calorie diets. Alternatives can be chosen from Calorie Tables (see Appendix), and Gordon's Diet Plan (p. 54) contains approximately 1,170 calories.

500 CALORIE DIET
(from Strang)

Protein 55 g.   *Carbohydrate* 40 g.   *Fat* 14 g.
Milk allowance: 10 oz. per day.
BREAKFAST
2 oz. cereal; 1 egg; 2 oz. fruit juice; milk from ration.
DINNER
3 oz. cottage cheese; 4 oz. vegetables; milk from ration.
SUPPER
$3\frac{1}{2}$ oz. meat or fish; 4 oz. vegetables; milk from ration.

1,000 CALORIE DIET   or   1,100 CALORIE DIET
(using skimmed milk)   (using ordinary milk)
Protein 60 g.   *Carbohydrate* 100 g.   *Fat* 40 g.
Milk Allowance: 10 oz. per day.
Butter Allowance: $\frac{1}{2}$ oz. per day.
BREAKFAST
1 orange or $\frac{1}{2}$ grapefruit; 1 oz. bread or 2 pieces Ryvita; 1 egg; milk and butter from ration.

DINNER
Clear soup; 2 to 3 oz. meat or fish; large helping of vegetables; 1 apple, pear or other fruit.

TEA
1 egg or $\frac{3}{4}$ oz. cheese or 1 oz. ham or tongue; fresh salad; 1 oz. bread.

SUPPER
1 oz. bread; butter and milk from ration; 1 orange.

BOOKS ON SLIMMING

A helpful book containing about 40 recipes suitable for slimmers is *Cooking for Special Diets* by Bee Nilson (Penguin, 7/6), and *The Slimmers Cook Book* by John Yudkin and Gweneth M. Chappell (Penguin, 4/6) gives interesting but expensive recipes. *The Slim Gourmet* by Martin Lederman (London, Oldbourne, 10/6) is full of useful tips for those who love their food, to enable them to enjoy quality rather than quantity.

REFERENCES

BANTING, W. (1864). *Letter on Corpulence*. London.
BLOOM, W. L. & CLARK, M. B. (1964). The obese carboholic. *J. Obesity*, **1**, 10.
CLEAVE, T. L. & CAMPBELL, G. D. (1966). *Diabetes, Coronary Thrombosis and the Saccharine Disease*. Bristol: Wright.
CHALMERS, T. H., KEKWICK, A. & PAWAN, G. L. S. (1958). On the fat mobilising activity of human urine. *Lancet*, **1**, 866.
CONSUMERS' ASSOCIATION (1967). *Which*. 10th Anniversary Issue 5th Oct.
DONALDSON, B. F. (1963). *Strong Medicine*. Cassell: London.
DUNCAN, L. J. P., ROSE, K. & MEIKLEJOHN, A. P. (1960). Phenmetrazine and methyl cellulose in the treatment of 'refractory' obesity. *Lancet*, **1**, 1262.
GORDON, E. S., GOLDBERG, M. & CHOSY, G. J. (1963). A new concept in the treatment of obesity. *J. Am. med. Ass.* **186**, 50.
HOWARD, A. N. & ANDERSON, T. B. (1968). The treatment of obesity with a high protein loaf. *Practitioner*, **201**, 491.
KEKWICK, A. & PAWAN, G. L. S. (1956). Calorie intake in relation to body weight changes in the obese. *Lancet*, **2**, 155.
KEKWICK, A. & PAWAN, G. L. S. (1964). The effects of high fat and high carbohydrate diets on rates of weight loss in mice. *Metabolism*, **13**, 87.
KEMP, R. (1966). Obesity as a disease. *Practitioner*, **196**, 404.
MARRIOTT, H. L. (1949). A simple weight reducing diet. *Br. med. J.* **2**, 18.
OLESON, E. S. & QUAADE, F. (1960). Fatty foods and obesity. *Lancet*, **1**, 1048.
PENNINGTON, A. W. (1951). The use of fat in a weight reducing diet. *Delaware St. med. J.* **23**, 79.
PILKINGTON, T. R., GAINSBOROUGH, H., ROSENOER, W. M. & CAREY, M. (1960). Diet and weight reduction in the obese. *Lancet*, **1**, 856.
RINZLER, S. H., ARCHER, M. & CHRISTAKIS, G. J. (1967). Primary prevention of coronary heart disease by diet. *Am. Heart J.* **73**, 287.
ROBERTS, H. J. (1964). The syndrome of narcolepsy and diabetogenic (functional) hyperinsulinism with special reference to obesity, diabetes, etc. *J. Am. Geriat. Soc.* **12**, 926.
SEATON, D. A. & ROSE, K. (1965). Defaulters from a weight reduction clinic. *J. chron. Dis.* **18**, 1007.
STRANG, J. M. (1964). *Disorders of Metabolism*. Ed. Duncan, G. G. 5th Ed. London: Saunders.
SILVERSTONE, J. T. & LOCKHEED, T. (1963). The value of a low carbohydrate diet in obese diabetics. *Metabolism*, **12**, 710.
WERNER, S. C. (1955). Comparison between weight reduction on a high calorie high fat diet and on an isocaloric regimen high in carbohydrates. *New Engl. J. Med.* **252**, 66.
YUDKIN, J. (1958). *This Slimming Business*. London: MacGibbon and Kee.
YUDKIN, J. & CAREY, M. (1960). The treatment of obesity by the high fat diet. *Lancet*, **2**, 939.

CHAPTER 7

The Treatment of Obesity by Drugs

ALL the drugs in common use in this country for the treatment of obesity belong to the group of anorexiants and there is no doubt that these drugs are effective in curbing appetite. Most of the drugs in controlled trials produce a substantially greater weight loss initially than the placebo, amounting usually to double the amount in the first two or three months. In most patients, however, the anorectic effect wears off after this time and after 12 months there may be no appreciable difference between the two groups. Silverstone & Solomon (1965) found that six out of 16 patients who completed a year on a placebo lost on average slightly more than five out of 12 who completed a year on diethylpropion although at three months the mean loss had been slightly less.

Patients lose weight more satisfactorily if they have been submitted to the discipline of dieting before being given an active drug. The results of two trials emphasise this point. Briggs, Newland & Bishop (1960) compared sixteen patients treated for a month by a 1,000 calorie diet and a placebo with 16 treated by the diet and phenmetrazine. For the second month the first group received phenmetrazine, and the second the placebo. Those who had received the drug first *gained* an average of 0·33 kg. (0·73 lb.) when on placebo in the second month, while those who had the placebo first lost 1·5 kg. (3·3 lb.) on it. The group who had the drug first lost an average of 2·6 kg. (5·8 lb.) in two months, while the group who had the placebo first, lost 4·4 kg. (9·7 lb.) in the two months. Brodbin & O'Connor (1967) using fenfluramine in 39 patients in general practice found that those who had used the drug first *gained* 1·07 kg. (2·37 lb.) on average on the placebo, while those using the placebo first lost 2·25 kg. (5·0 lb). Those who had the drug first lost a total of 8·75 (19·26 lb.) in the two months, and those who had the placebo first lost 6·67 kg. (14·75 lb.).

THE SIDE-EFFECTS OF ANOREXIANT DRUGS

As the side-effects of these drugs affect the doctor's decision as to which drug to use for a particular patient, these will now be considered.

All the effective drugs for curbing appetite belong to the amphetamine group, and there are three main types of side-effects.

1. *Those due to a stimulant effect upon the central nervous system.* These include nervousness and restlessness, irritability, insomnia, decreased sense of fatigue and euphoria, leading to **a danger of drug addiction.** See Case 5, page 69.

2. *Those due to a stimulation of the sympathetic nervous system (sympathomimetic).* These include dryness of the mouth, blurring of vision, light-headedness and dizziness, tachycardia and palpitations, elevation of the blood pressure and sweating.

3. *Those due to irritation of the gastro-intestinal tract.* These include nausea and vomiting, and constipation.

It should be noted that in controlled trials the incidence of this last group of ' side-effects ' is often as great when a placebo is being taken as when the active drug is being taken. Most of these side-effects must therefore be psychogenic in origin.

None of the sympathomimetic drugs should be used within 14 days of taking any of the mono-amine oxidase inhibitors, as severe hypertensive crises may occur.

The Council of the British Medical Association set up a Working Party in 1967 to investigate the usefulness or otherwise of amphetamine preparations. This Working Party recommended (1968) that ' amphetamines and amphetamine-like compounds should only be prescribed for those conditions for which no reasonable alternative exists, . . . more specifically (1) These drugs should be avoided so far as possible in the treatment of obesity, but if in individual cases the doctor feels they must be used they should be prescribed for a limited period only. Of the compounds available fenfluramine seems to have the least undesirable side-effects.' They also recommended that ' doctors should voluntarily take the same precautions and keep the same records as they already do for those drugs covered by Part I of the Schedule of the Dangerous Drugs Act, 1965.'

Comparisons of side-effects

Welsh, an American dermatologist with a special interest in obesity and a wide experience of the side-effects of anorectic drugs wrote a book in 1962 giving these side-effects in great detail. He used mainly diethylpropion, amphetamine and benzphetamine himself, but made an exhaustive search of the literature concerning the other anti-obesity drugs in general use at the time. He found diethylpropion to be slightly more efficient than the other drugs and in his series it showed a much lower instance of side-effects. Only 7 per cent of 752 patients had side-effects with diethylpropion compared with 33 per cent of 182 patients with benzphetamine and 35 per cent of 347 patients with amphetamine. *78 patients who had been unable to continue therapy with other anti-obesity drugs because of central nervous system effects were transferred to diethylpropion and were able to continue therapy.* 183 patients (24 per cent of the total) were kept on diethylpropion for periods of up to ten months and close supervision showed no evidence of dependence on medication.

Welsh mentions that 298 (40 per cent) of the patients on diethylpropion felt better while on the drug and he thinks that this may have been due to a slight degree of central nervous system stimulation. See also Table VI for the incidence of side-effects in general practice in this country. Diethylpropion gives the lowest incidence of the drugs reported.

REPORTS OF TREATMENT OF OBESITY BY DRUGS

Among hospital trials in the United Kingdom pride of place must go to Duncan and his team at The Royal Infirmary, Edinburgh, who conducted controlled trials between 1960 and 1968 on diethylpropion, chlorphentermine, dexamphetamine, fenfluramine and the biguanides. Silverstone, working from hospital, has organised trials with general practitioner colleagues (1956-67) on diethylpropion and Durophet M. Lorber working with children has compared dexamphetamine, phentermine and phenmetrazine, and many other hospital groups have reported results of treatment with one or more drugs.

There have been several series on the drug treatment of obesity published from general practice in the British Isles.

Fitzgerald & McElearney (1957) treated their patients with Filon, Jaffe (1961) treated 50 with diethylpropion, Smith (1962) 12 with phentermine, Reece (1963) 43 with diethylpropion, the General Practitioner Research Group (1961) 77 with chlorphentermine and 64 with Filon, Jackson & White (1965) 40 patients with chlorphentermine, Duncan *et al.* (1965) 78 with fenfluramine, Traherne (1967) 29 with fenfluramine, and Brodbin & O'Connor (1967) 39 with fenfluramine. Bew (1964) in a controlled trial compared dexamphetamine, benzphetamine, phenmetrazine and diethylpropion. Each agent was used until weight loss ceased when the patient was transferred to the next agent. He also used placebo tablets, known to him as such, when patients had lost the required amount of weight or if they showed signs of habituation to the drugs they were using. All patients were given a ' standard weight restricting diet '. In all, 34 patients lost an average of 4·5kg. (10 lb.) in nine weeks while on active drugs. The results were similar with each drug but patients stopped losing weight after an average of only 7 weeks on benzphetamine, compared with an average of 8½ weeks on diethylpropion, and 10½ weeks on dexamphetamine and phenmetrazine.

The results of drug therapy in the author's experience are summarised in Table V. In five years a total of 64 patients were given 158 courses of drugs.

Comparison between drugs

The main drugs that the author used each produced a similar degree of weight loss of approximately half a kilo or a pound a week for eight to 12 weeks. None of the recent general practice series in this country show an outstanding advantage for any drug in this respect, except perhaps for fenfluramine.

Walsh in his large series showed a better result with diethylpropion than with dexamphetamine or benzphetamine, but diethylpropion appeared to replace the other two in his therapeutic armamentarium and as the diethylpropion series is more recent than the other two it may be that the improved results were partly due to his increasing success in dealing with obese patients. Side effects are slightly less with diethylpropion than with dexamphetamine or phenmetrazine in the general practice series and are markedly less in Walsh's and the fact that he

TABLE V
Results of Drug Therapy in Author's Series

Drug	No. of Patients	Courses of treatment	Average weight loss kg. (lb.)	Side effects	Failed to lose wt.
Dexamphetamine	26	36	5·0 (11·0) in 8 weeks	5 (19%)	5
Phenmetrazine	33	51	4·3 (9·5) in 9½ weeks	7 (21%)	5
Diethylpropion	57	47	5·0 (11·0) in 10½ weeks	3 (8%)	5
Phentermine	9	13	3·4 (7·5) in 8 weeks	2 (22%)	1
Chlorphentermine	6	11	1·8 (4·0) in 6 weeks	2 (33%)	0
Total	111	158		19	16

TABLE VI
Summary of Results of Drug Therapy from General Practice Series 1961-1967

Drug	No. of patients	Average weight loss kg. (lb.)	Side effects	Failed to lose weight
Dexamphetamine	42	3·5 (8·5) in 8 weeks	7 (17%)	5 (12%)
Diethylpropion	182	5·2 (11·5) in 12 weeks	19 (10%)	17 (9%)
Phenmetrazine	46	4·1 (9·0) in 9 weeks	9 (19%)	5 (11%)
Phentermine	21	4·75 (10·5) in 11 weeks	2 (10%)	2 (10%)
Chlorphentermine	77	4·1 (9·0) in 13 weeks	26 (33%)	11 (14%)
Fenfluramine	146	4·1 (9·0) in 6 weeks	27 (18%)	?

found no evidence of drug dependence in 184 cases is a strong point in favour of diethylpropion compared with the other major drugs. Nevertheless a case has been reported of addiction to diethylpropion (Clein & Benady, 1962) and care must still be taken with it.

Diethylpropion appears to be at least as efficacious as the other major anorectics and to have a lesser tendency to produce side-effects. In spite of its price therefore diethylpropion appears to be the drug of choice.

Method of administering drugs

Many drugs are available in short acting and long acting forms. Ion exchange resins, which are the form in which most of the long acting anorectic agents are presented, provide dependable sustained release oral medication superior to other forms of long acting preparation, as only one factor affects their release, whereas other forms are affected by up to nine different factors (Sensenbach & Hays, 1966). The advantage of the short acting form is that a patient is reminded of his diet by taking a tablet before meals, whereas the long acting form prevents a sudden access of hunger during the day, is ideal for the patient who is likely to forget to take a second or third tablet, and is probably the most suitable form for general use.

Continuous or intermittent therapy?

Munro *et al.* (1968) in Edinburgh compared phentermine given continuously with phentermine alternated with a dummy capsule every month for a total of nine months. With both methods of treatment a steady loss of weight of over 0·45 kg. (1 lb.) per week continued for five or six months in over half of those who commenced the trial. They have made a strong case for alternating treatment with placebo on grounds of cost and safety. Dummy capsules are not available for general use, but a placebo such as a small dose of a tranquilliser in tense patients would seem to be a useful alternative.

Le Riche & Csima (1967) in Toronto did a similar trial with diethylpropion, and obtained a better weight loss with those on continuous therapy, but only 14 out of 99 on continuous therapy and 22 out of 101 on intermittent therapy completed six months, so that further trials of this sort are obviously necessary.

THE INDICATIONS FOR DRUG THERAPY

The author gives drugs in the following circumstances:

1. To enable a co-operative patient to continue to keep strictly to a diet once the initial motivation has worn off.

2. As a temporary expedient from the beginning of treatment in certain depressed patients, and patients with peptic ulcer who have difficulty in keeping to a diet.

3. In short courses at six monthly or yearly intervals to enable patients to regain a more normal weight after having relapsed, and in certain cases of relapse following previous loss of weight where the patient had difficulty in keeping to a diet.

4. In patients who had failed to lose weight on a diet.

The last indication might appear to be a doubtful one as none of the patients achieved a satisfactory and permanent weight loss, but those achieving intermittent weight loss might progress to a greater weight if they were not helped to lose weight occasionally. See Case 3, page 69.

The use of drugs for periods longer than three months

Seven of the author's patients took drugs for 20 to 30 weeks under strict supervision and the drug was stopped in all cases when the rate of loss of weight diminished. They lost an average of 17·2 kg. (38 lb.) in 20 weeks. An eighth patient was not strictly supervised and gained 2·7 kg. (6 lb.) in 69 weeks. Details of some of these patients follow:

CASE 1: Mrs. E. can only be saved from gross obesity by regular courses of drugs. She is childless and enjoys her food. On one occasion she took phenmetrazine for 26 weeks and had lost 17·2 kg. (38 lb.) when she ceased attending.

CASE 2: Mrs. D., aged 62 (followed up for $4\frac{3}{4}$ years) put on 13·6 kg. (30 lb.) weight following an arthrodesis to her left knee. She had previously dieted with some success, but now asked for help with drugs to enable her to mobilise quickly. In the course of 21 weeks on diethylpropion she lost steadily to a total of 13·1 kg. (29 lb.) but during the sixth month she lost only 0·45 kg. (1 lb.). She was asked to try for a month without any medication and during this time she lost a further 2·7 kg. (6 lb.). This suggests that she had come to rely on the drug to the exclusion of diet for her weight reduction. On losing the habit of taking the drug she dieted more strictly with satisfactory results.

CASE 3: Miss F., aged 38 is mentally subnormal. She was anxious to become less stout, but could not diet without help; her initial weight was 68·8 kg. (152 lb.). She lost 10·5 kg. (23 lb.) in 13 weeks with phenmetrazine, and a further 3·2 kg. (7 lb.) in the next 10 weeks (a total of 20 per cent of her initial weight) and was approaching her normal weight. The drug was then stopped. One year later she had maintained her weight loss, but after two further years had regained a little over half of it.

CASE 4: This is Case No. 6 in the Children's series (p. 168). Miss G., at the age of 17 and a weight of 102 kg. (225·5 lb.) suddenly decided to take an interest in her appearance. She lost 7·5 kg. (16·5 lb.) in 10 weeks with diethylpropion, put on 1·6 kg. (3·5 lb.) in one week on changing to fenfluramine, and after battling for a few months with occasional help from diethylpropion again, decided to give it up because her nights were becoming restless. That this was probably not a true drug effect is shown by the fact that she ' cured her insomnia by taking one aspirin nightly.' She commenced successful dieting after a break of only two weeks, losing 3·2 kg. (7 lb.) in two weeks with diethylpropion, and then on changing to chlorphentermine lost a total of 25·8 kg. (57 lb.) in 30 weeks (total loss 37·8 kg. (83·5 lb.) over a period of 60 weeks). She had been seen fortnightly throughout, and had lost weight at each visit except on the occasion when she changed to fen-fluramine

CASE 5: Mrs. H. (No. 6 in group 4) lost 5·4 kg (12 lb.) in 18 weeks on diet alone. Four years later she had relapsed, but lost 3·6 kg. (8 lb.) in seven weeks on phenmetrazine. The author lost sight of her personally for the next sixteen months and found that during that time she had been given eleven repeat prescriptions of 30 days' supply by a colleague, during which time she had put on 2·7 kg. (6 lb.) and was almost back to where she had started. A widow, she was working full-time to keep her only child at school during this period. Fortunately, she did not become addicted and is now keeping her weight stationary without drugs, but the careless prescription of this drug could very well have led to addiction in a less stable personality.

It follows from these cases that **no patient should be given drugs for longer than three months save in very exceptional circumstances, and the utmost vigilance should be exercised in supervision throughout.** No patient should be given a prescription for anorectic drugs without seeing their doctor and being weighed.

DRUGS USED FOR WEIGHT REDUCTION

Details are appended concerning all the drugs in common use in Great Britain and the U.S.A.

Anorectics: (a) the amphetamine group, (b) methylamphetamine, (c) phenmetrazine and phendimetrazine, (d) phenbutrazate, (e) diethylpropion, (f) phentermine, (g) chlorphentermine, (h) benzphetamine and (i) fenfluramine.

Oral Hypoglycaemic agents: (a) phenformin and (b) metformin.

Metabolic stimulators: i.e. the thyroid group of drugs.

Laxatives.

ANORECTICS

The Amphetamine Group

The Dextro-rotary isomer has replaced amphetamine itself for clincal use in the treatment of obesity. The laevo rotary isomer, although not so powerful with its anorectic effect, is also used.

Proprietary Products	Manufacturer	Preparation
Dexamed	Medo	Tabs. D-amphetamine Sulph. 5 mg.
		Also Amphedase and Amplus (U.S.A.)
Dexten	Nicholas	Tabs. D-amphetamine Resinate 10 mg.
Dexedrine	S. K. & F.	Sustained release Spansules. D-amphet. Sulph. 10 mg. 15 mg.
		Also Dadex Timules, D-Ate. Caps. (U.S.A.)
Bontid	Carnick	Carboxymethylcellulose Salt of D-amphetamine 5 mg.
Levenor	Genatosan	L-amphetamine Alginate 5 mg.
		Also Cydril Laevomine (U.S.A.)
* Durophet	Riker	Caps. D-amphet. Resinate 3 parts, L-amphetamine 1 part. 7·5 mg. 12·5 mg. 20 mg.

Combined with sedatives

Barbidex	Nicholas	Tabs. D-amphet. Resinate 10 mg., Phenobarbitone 30 mg.
*Durophet M	Riker	L and D-amphet. Resinates 12·5 mg. 20 mg. Methaqualone 40 mg.
Appetrol	Wallace	D-amphet. Sulph. 5 mg. Meprobamate 400 mg.
Steladex	S. K. & F.	Sustained release Spansules. D-amphet. 10 mg. Tripluoperazine 2 mg.

Also Amodex, Bemadex, Dexamyl, Dexatal Dura-tabs, Eskatrol, Rauwiarine, Thora-Dex, Vita Respital, Bontril, Amplus with Atarax, Seco-Synatan (U.S.A.).

* Category B.1. Proplist 1968.

The amphetamine group were in use for almost ten years before other sympathomimetic anorectic drugs, so that they form the obvious standard of comparison for the others.

DOSE. 5-30 mg. daily in divided dose or sustained action.

SIDE-EFFECTS. *C.S.N. stimulation*—Restlessness and irritability 23 per cent of 347 patients (Welsh), insomnia 15 per cent of 347 patients (Welsh), euphoria and elation, lessened sense of fatigue.

Fatigue and depression may follow the temporary mental stimulation. Large doses can lead to addiction and to toxic psychosis, but there are wide variations in response to the drug.

Sympathomimetic effects—pressor response to ephedrine potentiate. Raised blood pressure 8 per cent (Welsh), dryness of the mouth 13 per cent (Welsh), dizziness 9 per cent (Welsh), diuresis, sweating.

CONTRA-INDICATIONS. Hypertension, coronary artery disease. Anxiety. Unstable personality.

EFFECTIVENESS. It is equal in effect to most of its successors. D-amphet. resinate is likely to be the best preparation as there is less chance of rebound of fatigue and depression when the effect wears off (Abrahams & Linnell 1957, Lorber 1966).

ASSESSMENT. The cheapest of all the agents, amphetamine is very variable in its effects and is prone to lead to addiction unless carefully controlled. Three cases of addiction to d-amphetamine sulphate have come under the author's care, although none were initiated by its use as an anorectic. The danger is nevertheless always present. *As the effect is so variable in the individual it is doubtful whether it should ever be used except in patients who have had it previously without detriment.*

METHYLAMPHETAMINE

Proprietary Product	Manu- facturer	Preparation
Metamsustac	Pharmax	Sustained action tablets 7·5 mg. 15 mg.
Desbutal	Abbott	Caps. { Methlyamphetamine 5 mg. Pentobarbitone Na. 30 mg.

SIDE-EFFECTS. In Welsh's series of 194 patients these were *similar to those produced by amphetamine, but with a higher proportion of C.N.S. stimulating effects.*

EFFECTIVENESS. Similar to amphetamine.

ASSESSMENT. No indications for use.

PHENMETRAZINE HCl

Proprietary Product	*Manu-facturer*	*Preparation*
Preludin	Boehringer	Tabs. 25 mg.
		Sustained action tabs. (Tablongets) 50 mg.

FIRST USED. Germany, 1954; U.S.A., 1956; Great Britain, 1958.

DOSE. 25 mg. b.d. or t.d.s.
50 mg. Tablonget 1 or 2 mane.

SIDE-EFFECTS. *C.N.S. stimulation.* Restlessness, irritability, euphoria, aggressiveness.

Sympathomimetic. Dry mouth, blurring of vision, palpitations, elevation of the blood pressure. 25 (6·4 per cent) out of 392 patients had to stop treatment because of side-effects on a daily dose of 30 mg. (Bienart & Ueberla, 1967).

All side effects are less common with the long acting preparation and are usually reduced by modifying the dosage. Insomnia is rarely a problem but it is wise to give the last dose not later than 4 p.m. at first. Cases of *psychosis* and *addiction* were reported before phenmetrazine was put on Schedule 4. Cases of addiction were reported by Bethel (1957) and Silverman (1959). Evans (1959) reported 12 cases of psychosis seen by him in six months.

EFFECTIVENESS. Rendle-Short (1960) found that 21 children who were not put on a diet lost an average of 1·4 kg. (3·1 lb.) in four weeks, while with a placebo an increase of weight averaging 0·75 kg. (1·7 lb.) occurred in the same period. With the long acting form Howard *et al.* (1964) secured a weight loss in 59/60 patients averaging 8·5 kg. (18·8 lb.) in an average of 9·6 weeks. None of these had to stop treatment on account of side effects. In comparison with other agents phenmetrazine can hold its own and in the author's hands has been comparable with dexamphetamine and diethylpropion (Table V).

CONTRA-INDICATION. Hypertension or acute coronary disease.

ASSESSMENT. Phenmetrazine has stood the test of time as an effective agent with a minimum of side effects, especially in the long acting form. It may be the anorectic of choice in obese diabetics (p. 176). The Tablonget is recommended for patients who are lethargic and in whom a mild stimulant effect is desirable.

PHENDIMETRAZINE

This is marketed as Plegine in the U.S.A. but not in this country; it has a similar action to phenmetrazine but is stated to have less pressor effects.

PHENMETRAZINE THEOCLATE 20 mg.

PHENBUTRAZATE HCl 30 mg.

The two drugs are said to act antagonistically on the autonomic nervous system so that there is no significant effect on the blood pressure or heart rate.

Phenbutrazate HCl

Phenmetrazine formula—page 72

FIRST USED. Germany, 1955 (under the name of Califon as a mild central stimulant in cases of tuberculosis, but it was later used for appetite control); Great Britain, 1957 (Fitzgerald & McElearney).

DOSE. 50 mg. twice daily increased up to eight times daily if necessary. No dose should be taken after 4 p.m.

SIDE-EFFECTS. Usually mild consisting of vertigo, restlessness, palpitations and insomnia. In the General Practitioner Research Group series (1961) five cases out of 64 had to stop treatment on account of side effects.

EFFECTIVENESS. Weight loss during the first six weeks of therapy is greater than placebo. Average weight lost 0·8 kg. (1·8 lb.) weekly for eight weeks (G.P.R.G., 1961).

ASSESSMENT. There have been no control trials against other anorectic agents, but there appear to be no outstanding advantages of this combination in comparison with phenmetrazine alone, to justify the extra cost.

Diethylpropion HCl

$$
\underset{\text{CH}_3}{\underset{|}{\text{C}_6\text{H}_5}-\overset{\overset{\text{O}}{\|}}{\text{C}}-\text{CH}-\text{N}.\text{HCl}.}
$$

(structure: benzene ring — C(=O) — CH(CH₃) — N.HCl with two C₂H₅ substituents)

Proprietary Product	Manufacturer	Preparation
Apisate	Wyeth	Tabs. { diethylpropion HCl. 75 mg. / Vitamin B. group
Tenuate	Merrill	Tabs. diethylpropion HCl. 25 mg.
Tenuate Dospan	do.	Sustained action tabls. 75 mg.

This is a sympathomimetic amine with a much lower incidence of side-effects due to C.N.S. stimulation than the other members of the group.

FIRST USED. U.S.A, 1959; Great Britain, 1961 (Jaffe; Seaton *et al.*).

DOSE. 1 or 2 sustained action tablets in the morning, or 3 to 4 25 mg. tablets daily, not later than 6 p.m.

SIDE-EFFECTS. *C.N.S. stimulation.* Less than 1 per cent in Walsh's large series of 752 patients, drowsiness: 1 per cent, felt more relaxed: 4 per cent.

Sympathomimetic. Occasionally experienced, including dryness of the mouth. Rare cases of *addiction* have been reported. In Clein and Benady's case (1962) the patient had previously been addicted to dexamphetamine and phenmetrazine.

EFFECTIVENESS. Walsh (1962) found diethylpropion to be slightly more effective than amphetamine and benzphetamine, but as it replaced the other drugs he may have become more expert in the treatment of obesity. Bew (1964) in general practice found no appreciable difference between dexamphetamine, phenmetrazine and diethylpropion and findings in the author's practice were similar (Table V).

ASSESSMENT. Diethylpropion is equally as effective as other agents and has a lower incidence of side-effects, in particular those associated with C.N.S. stimulation. Oswald *et al.* (1968) have shown that the depth of sleep is lightened compared with a placebo and in this respect it is inferior to fenfluramine, but as pointed out by Silverstone (1968) he gave *two* tablets ' 1 to $1\frac{1}{2}$ hours before lights out ' whereas in clinical practice *one* tablet is given about 6 p.m. to give the maximum clinical effect in the evening. Silverstone & Clery (1967) showed that under strict double blind controlled conditions diethylpropion did not significantly or materially alter the quality of sleep reported by the patients.

Diethlypropion in the long acting form appears to be the agent of first choice for most cases of obesity.

PHENTERMINE

Proprietary Product	Manufacturer	Preparation
Duromine	Ricker	Caps. Phentermine Resin 15 mg. and 30 mg.

FIRST USED. U.S.A., 1959; Great Britain, 1962 (Smith).

DOSE. One 15 mg. or 30 mg. caps. before breakfast.

SIDE-EFFECTS. *C.N.S. stimulation.* Less than with amphetamine itself.

Sympathomimetic. Dry mouth the most common.

EFFECTIVENESS. Equal to its competitors in general practice trials in this country, including the author's small experience. Munro *et al.* (1968) used it for their comparison of continuous and intermittent therapy and produced a steady fall of weight for about five months averaging over 0·4 kg. (1 lb.) per week by both methods in 39/72 patients who completed the trial.

ASSESSMENT. A useful alternative to diethylpropion especially where the capsule form of medication has psychological advantages.

CHLORPHENTERMINE HCl

Proprietary Product	Manufacturer	Preparation
Lucofen S.A.	Warner	75 mg. sustained release tablets.
Pre-Sate (U.S.A.)	do.	

FIRST USED. Great Britain, 1960; U.S.A., 1965.

DOSE. One or two tablets of 75 mg. daily.

SIDE-EFFECTS. Less C.N.S. side-effects than with amphetamine. Dryness of the mouth, nausea, dizziness and headache. Eight of 77 patients omitted treatment because of the side-effects (G.P.R.G., 1960) with uncoated short acting tablets.

EFFECTIVENESS. Average loss per week for 71 patients was 0·5 kg. (1·1 lb.) (G.P.R.G., 1961). In a refractory group of 30 women at least 20 per cent overweight, average loss was 0·32 kg. (0·7 lb.) per week for 6 weeks (Seaton *et al.*, 1964). In 40 patients at least 20 per cent overweight, average loss per week was 0·64 kg. (1·42 lb.) for 4 weeks (Jackson & White, 1965).

ASSESSMENT. Chlorphentermine appears as effective as other agents of the same group and has less C.N.S. side-effects than all except diethylpropion and fenfluramine. A useful alternative.

BENZPHETAMINE HCl

Proprietary Product	Manufacturer	Preparation
Didrex	Upjohn	Tablets 25 mg.

FIRST USED. U.S.A., 1960; United Kingdom, 1964.

DOSE. 1 to 3 of the 25 mg. tablets daily, but as much as 450 mg. a day has been used in resistant cases (Kay *et al.*, 1961).

SIDE-EFFECTS. *C.N.S. stimulation.* This occurs in a small proportion even on a small dosage (three out of 29 in Bew's series).

Sympathomimetic. Palpitations, dry mouth and dizziness as well as nausea occur occasionally. Walsh (1962) found that side effects occurred about as frequently as with amphetamine with a dose of 50 to 100 mg. daily.

EFFECTIVENESS, Walsh, who used it in 182 cases, found it to be *approximately equal to amphetamine.* In the series studied by Kay *et al.* (1961) 46 out of 50 lost an average of 0·4 kg. (0·9 lb.) per week for an average time of 16 weeks. In Bew's series (1964) six patients lost an average of 0·7 kg. (1·5 lb.) per week for an average of seven weeks before weight loss ceased, but patients on D-amphetamine, phenmetrazine and diethylpropion continued to lose weight for an average of 10 weeks, so that benzphetamine may be slightly less effective than the others.

ASSESSMENT. It has no particular advantage to offer over any of its competitors, and has not established itself in the British market.

FENFLURAMINE

Remains present in the body for a long time on account of its considerable tissue fixation, particularly in the fatty tissues.

Proprietary Product	Manufacturer	Preparation
Ponderax	Selpharm Labs.	Tablets 20 mg.

FIRST USED. France, 1963. First trial results 1965 after 600 patients had used the drug for two years (Lambusier, 1965). General practice trials in Great Britain, Duncan *et. al.* (1965), Traherne (1965), Brodbin & O'Connor (1967).

DOSE. Two or three long acting 20 mg. tablets daily. Usually given mid-morning and tea-time, but dose can be increased to four or five daily if necessary.

TOXICITY. No fatalities have been reported even with overdoses of 80 and 90 tablets respectively (White *et al.*, 1967).

SIDE-EFFECTS. None attributable to C.N.S. stimulation in most cases. This clinical impression has been confirmed by the absence of critical flicker frequency (Hill & Turner, 1967). They say that this method is a valuable test of central function which has been shown to be sensitive in assessing the action of several centrally acting drugs. Nevertheless, the depth of sleep is lightened compared with a placebo (Oswald *et al.*, 1968). However, fenfluramine is superior in this respect to diethylpropion, which was previously the anorectic with the least stimulant effect on the C.N.S. *Sedation* is the commonest side effect, but is usually abolished by a reduction of dosage. It occurred in 13 per cent of Duncan's 78 cases (three or four tablets daily) and in three out of 39 (7·8 per cent) of Brodbin & O'Connor's patients on a dosage of two tablets daily. Other side-effects are mild and unimportant. Diarrhoea, dry mouth, dizziness, nausea and headache have been reported. There is no effect on the blood pressure.

EFFECTIVENESS. The short term effects bear comparison with any of its predecessors. Brodbin & O'Connor's patients averaged 0·86 kg. (1·9 lb.) loss per week for six weeks, compared with ·09 kg. (0·2 lb.) per week for placebo in a double blind trial (1,000 cal. diet) and Duncan *et al.* found that 78 patients averaged 1 kg. (2·2 lb.) per week for four weeks compared with 0·5 kg. (1·1 lb.) per week on placebo (low C.H. diet). Spence & Medvei (1967) found it to be effective in 20 out of 33 patients. In 18 patients, compared with sustained action d-amphet-sulph. it was more effective in 10 and equal in a further four.

LONG-TERM EFFECTS. In most subjects the drug appears to retain its effect beyond the usual six to eight weeks of its competitors (Munro, Seaton & Duncan, 1966). This may be due to a direct effect on metabolism (p. 39).

Comparison with other agents. Munro, Seaton & Duncan (1966) comparing fenfluramine with drugs used in previous trials at the same clinic under similar conditions, found it to be superior to phenmetrazine, diethylpropion, chlorphentermine, dexamphetamine and phentermine, but further comparative trials are necessary before its place is clearly outlined.

ASSESSMENT. This is the preparation of choice for patients who are tense and anxious, and if initial trial results are confirmed it may possibly supersede diethylpropion as the preparation of choice for most patients.

THE COST OF ANORECTIC DRUGS
See Table VII

The price to the nation of a drug varies with the size of the pack from which the chemist takes his supply. To the minimum basic price from a large pack as shown in M.I.M.S. has been added $10\frac{1}{2}$ per cent together with 2s 3d as the chemist's professional fee and 2d container fee, to produce the minimum cost to the nation.

ORAL HYPOGLYCAEMIC AGENTS

PHENFORMIN HCl (DIBOTIN)

$$\langle \text{ring} \rangle - CH_2 - CH_2 - NH - \underset{\underset{NH}{\parallel}}{C} - NH - \underset{\underset{NH}{\parallel}}{C} - NH_2$$

Phenformin causes weight loss in a higher proportion of obese diabetics than other oral hypoglycaemic compounds. In some obese non-diabetics who have a raised plasma insulin level and show a hypoglycaemic response to glucose due to insulin resistance, this insulin resistance is abolished by phenformin in the same way as it is in obese diabetics (p. 39). It

TABLE VII

Total Minimum Cost of Prescribing Two Weeks' Supply of Drugs in the Usual Dosage

Proprietary Preparation	No. of Tablets	Total Cost to Nearest 1d at 1st January, 1969
Apisate	14	6s 5d.
Appetrol	42	11s. 3d.
Appetrol S.R.	14	7s. 7d.
Barbidex	14	4s. 4d.
Desbutal	42	6s. 3d.
Dexamed	42	4s. 0d.
Dexamphetamine Sulph. 5 mg.	42	2s 10d.
Dexedrine Spansules 10 mg.	14	4s. 6d.
Dexedrine Spansules 15 mg.	14	4. 11d.
Dexten	14	3s. 8d.
Didrex	42	8s. 2d.
Duromine 15 mg.	14	6s. 4d.
Duromine 30 mg.	14	6s. 10d.
Durophet 7·5	14	3s. 6d.
Durophet 12·5	14	3s. 8d.
Durophet 20	14	4s. 0d.
Durophet M 12·5	14	4s. 8d.
Durophet M 20	14	4s. 11d.
Filon	42	12s. 7d.
Lucofen S.A.	14	6s. 9d.
Metamsustac 7·5	14	4s. 7d.
Metamsustac 15	14	4s. 11d.
Ponderax	28	13s. 2d.
Preludin 25 mg.	42	8s. 9d.
Preludin tablongets 50 mg.	14	7s. 1d.
Steladex sp.	14	9s. 6d.
Tenuate	42	9s. 5d.
Tenuate Dospan	14	6s. 3d.

therefore seems reasonable to suppose that weight loss could
be produced by phenformin in these subjects by reversing this
abnormal metabolic tendency.

Roginsky & Barnett (1966) gave 14 obese non-diabetic
subjects two 50 mg. timed-disintegration capsules of phenformin daily for 15 weeks, and a comparable group of 13
subjects identical placebo capsules for the same time. All
were on a 1,000 calorie low-carbohydrate diet. Six patients
with a family history of diabetes lost an average of 12 kg.
(26·5 lb.) with phenformin compared with an average of 4·3 kg.
(9·4 lb.) for those with no family history. The four subjects
with a diabetic family history lost only 5·8 kg. (12·8 lb.) on
the placebo and the nine subjects without a family history
lost an average of 5 kg. (11·0 lb.). Thus those patients with
a close family history of diabetes lost over twice as much
weight on phenformin as those with no such history, the latter
losing approximately the same weight as the patients on the
placebo.

Duncan and his colleagues in Edinburgh (Munro *et al.*,
1968) showed in a double-blind controlled trial lasting for 16
weeks that both phenformin and metformin caused significant
weight loss in women suffering from ' refractory obesity '.
An average of 3·3 kg. (7·3 lb.) was lost by 24 patients on phenformin, 26 on metformin lost an average of 2·9 kg. (6·5 lb.)
while 27 patients on placebos *gained* an average of 1·9 kg.
(2·6 lb.). In the two drug series there was no difference between
the group of 15 women with a strong family history of diabetes
or who had had a 4·5 kg. (10 lb.) baby, and the remaining 35
women. It is likely, however, that these 35 women having
attended the Obesity Clinic for at least one year without
benefit, had all been overweight long enough to have developed
insulin resistance which the drugs were capable of abolishing.
In this series the dose of drug was pushed until gastric intolerance showed itself or until 300 mg. phenformin or 3,000 mg.
metformin daily were being taken. The dose of phenformin
averaged 200 mg. per day and that of metformin 2,500 mg.
per day. On breaking down the series, approximately half on
each drug (14 out of 24 on phenformin and 12 out of 26 on
metformin) lost at least 3·6 kg. (8 lb.) in 16 weeks, but in
several cases the drug had to be continued for six weeks or

longer before a loss of 1·3 kg. (3 lb.) was achieved as it often took several weeks to reach the optimum dosage.

DOSAGE. Two sustained release 50 mg. capsules daily increasing by one capsule daily each week until gastric irritation occurs or 6 capsules daily are taken.

ASSESSMENT. More expensive than metformin (q.v.).

It is not practicable to obtain plasma insulin levels for ordinary clinical purposes, so that on clinical grounds it would appear reasonable to use phenformin in two groups of obese persons:

1. Those with a close family history of diabetes.
2. Those who have been persistently overweight for a long period (say 10 years) and have been 'refractory' to normal methods of treatment.

The author gave phenformin to five women who had been obese for 20 years or more. Two stopped treatment because of nausea, one lost no weight after 9 weeks, one lost only 1·4 kg. (3 lb.) in six weeks but felt fitter than she had done for years, and the other lost 8·6 kg. (19 lb.) in 13 weeks to reach her lowest weight for 18 years.

METFORMIN HCl. (GLUCOPHAGE)

This is a biguinide, like phenformin:

$$(CH_3)_2 - N - \overset{\overset{\displaystyle NH}{\|}}{C} - NH - \overset{\overset{\displaystyle NH}{\|}}{C} - NH_2$$

Like phenformin it causes weight loss in many obese diabetics. It can be used in some non-obese diabetics in the same way as phenformin (q.v.).

DOSAGE. Two 500 mg. tablets daily increasing by one tablet daily each week until gastric irritation occurs or six tablets daily are taken.

ASSESSMENT. Cheaper than phenformin and possibly therefore the agent of first choice in refractory obesity of long standing, or where there is a close family history of obesity.

METABOLIC STIMULATORS

THYROID AND ITS ANALOGUES

Tri-iodothyronine

HO$-$⬡$_I$$-O-$⬡$-CH_2$$-$ CH $-$ COOH with I substituents, and NH$_2$ below CH

Thyroxine

HO$-$⬡$-$O$-$⬡$-$CH$_2$$-$ CH $-$ COOH with I substituents, and NH$_2$ below CH

Tri-iodothyronine is the precursor of thyroid hormone and according to Goodman & Gilman (1965) acts more rapidly than thyroxine, which acts more rapidly than thyroid. They state that there is no significant difference in the response of the patient with myxoedema to these substances. The normal daily maintenance doses in myxoedema are: thyroid, 120-180 mg., thyroxine, 0·1-0·2 mg., tri-iodothyronine, 25-75 μg.

There has recently been a revival of the use of thyroid, thyroxine and tri-iodothyronine in the U.S.A. and on the continent, using doses much larger than the physiological ones. Of 200 obese patients seen by Roberts in Miami, U.S.A. (1964) 33 had been taking thyroid or tri-iodothyronine before coming under his care.

Kyle *et al.* (1966) used 30 to 180 mg. of thyroid daily in two cases of myxoedema and found that loss of fat was only 39 and 31 per cent: in two cases of obesity they gave doses of 300 to 900 mg. (5-15 grains) thyroid daily and found that weight loss was increased, but the loss was mainly of protein and only 30 to 40 per cent of fat.

Gordon (1963) found that the defective free fatty acid mobilisation by l-epinephine (adrenaline) was corrected by tri-iodothyronine, but not by thyroxine or desiccated thyroid. Tri-iodothyronine was also found to increase glucose oxidation in those individuals in whom the rate had previously been decreased. Kneebone (1966) used it successfully in obese children.

This theoretical advantage of tri-iodothyronine over thyroxine found by Gordon was not shown to lead to any clinical difference in a controlled trial by Gwinup & Poucher (1967) who put alternate obese patients on the drugs without any dietary restrictions, gradually increasing the dose until signs of nervousness or tachycardia appeared and then reducing it. Of 17 patients two withdrew because of nervous symptoms and two, both with a positive family history of diabetes, because of glycosuria; six patients completed 30 weeks with tri-iodothyronine and lost an average of 11·3 kg. (25 lb.) on an average dose of 275 μg. daily while the seven patients on thyroxine lost an average of 13·6 kg. (30 lb.) on an average dose of 1,400 μg. daily On stopping treatment the weight returned rapidly to normal. Four patients on placebo tablets gained an average of over 2·25 kg. (5 lb.) in 13 weeks and were removed from the study due to their discontent at failure to lose weight. The author's comment ' the use of therapeutic doses of thyroid analogs . . . merely substitutes one clinical entity for another (thyrotoxicosis for obesity) '.

ASSESSMENT. The induction of thyrotoxicosis in obese subjects may be dangerous, especially in subjects with occult coronary athero-sclerosis, and it would appear that as the loss of weight consists mainly of protein and only persists while the drugs are being given, this treatment should only be used for research purposes at present.

LAXATIVES

These are included in several proprietary brands of slimming tablets (Obesettes for example) and presumably produce a slight initial weight loss owing to loss of fluid. In almost every case some sort of dietary advice is included in the packaging. Laxatives have been shown conclusively to be ineffective agents in weight reduction by Bienert & Ueberla (1967) who compared phenmetrazine with a tablet containing a laxative in addition to the same drug. In a very thorough controlled trial there was no difference in effect between the two preparations.

NEW DRUGS AND THE FUTURE

The control of obesity by drugs is unlikely to lie in the field of better anorexiants, as it is difficult to envisage an anorectic drug being produced which has any major advantage over those in use at present. Promising avenues of approach are the oral hypoglycaemic agents for the patient with long-standing obesity; fenfluramine or a derivative for its metabolic effect if the increased glucose uptake by muscle is confirmed in a larger group of patients; and ' fat mobilising hormone ' or some substance similar in action to it which would be effective for all patients (p. 27).

REFERENCES

ABRAHAM, Sir Adolphe & LINNELL, W. H. (1957). Oral depot therapy with a new long-acting detamphetamine salt. *Lancet,* **2,** 1317.
BETHEL, M. F. (1957). Toxic psychosis caused by ' Preludin '. *Br. med. J.* **1,** 30.
BEW, K. (1964). A study of obesity in general practice. *Ulster med. J.* **33,** 43.
BIENART, H. R. & UEBERLE, K. (1967). Therapeutic testing of an anorectic agent (Preludin Compound). *Arzneimittel-Forsch.* **17,** 336.
BRIGGS, J. H., NEWLAND, P. M. & BISHOP, P. M. F. (1960). Phenmetrazine hydrochloride in treatment of obesity. *Br. med. J.* **2,** 911.
BRITISH MEDICAL ASSOCIATION WORKING PARTY (1968). Control of amphetamine preparations. *Br. med. J.* **2,** 572.
BRODBIN, P. & O'CONNOR, C. A. (1967). A double-blind clinical trial of an appetite depressant, fenfluramine, in general practice. *Practitioner,* **198,** 707.
CLEIN, L. D. & BENADY, D. R. (1962). Case of diethylpropion addiction. *Br. med. J.* **2,** 450.
COUNCIL ON DRUGS (1966). Chlorphentermine hydrochloride. *J. Am. med. Ass.* **196,** 165.
DUHOULT, J. & FENARD, S. (1965). Investigation of the excretion, localisation and metabolism of a new anorectic substance: fenfluramine. *Archs int. Pharmacodyn. Thér.* **158,** 1.
DUNCAN, E. H., HYDE, C. A., REGAN, N. A. & SWEETMAN, B. (1965). A preliminary trial of fenfluramine in general practice. *Br. J. clin. Pract.* **19,** 451.
DUNCAN, L. J. P. & MUNRO, J. F. (1968). The present status of anorexiant drugs. *Practitioner,* **200,** 167.
EVANS, J. (1959). Psychosis and addiction to phenmetrazine. *Lancet,* **2,** 152.

FINEBERG, S. K. (1961). Obesity, diabetes and anorexigenics. *J. Am. med. Ass.* **175**, 680.

FINEBERG, S. K. (1966). Diabetes—obesity: a new concept and its management. *Md med. J.* **15**, 39.

FITZGERALD, O. & McELEARNEY, L. G. (1957). Clinical trial of Cafilon and Ritalin in the treatment of obesity. *Ir. J. med. Sci.* **381**, 391.

GENERAL PRACTITIONER RESEARCH GROUP (1961). Lucofen trial. *Practitioner,* **187**, 216.

GOODMAN, L. S. & GILMAN, A. (1965). *The Pharmacological Basis of Therapeutics.* 3rd Ed. New York: Macmillan.

GWINUP, G. & POUCHER, R. (1967). A controlled study of thyroid analogs in the therapy of obesity. *Am. J. med. Sci.* **50**, 416.

HAMPSON, J., LORAINE, J. A. & STRONG, J. A. (1960). Phenmetrazine and dexamphetamine in the management of obesity. *Lancet,* **1**, 1265.

HILL, R. C. & TURNER, P. (1967). Fenfluramine and critical flicker frequency. *J. Pharm. Pharmac.* **19**, 337.

JACKSON, I. M. D. & WHYTE, W. G. (1965). Chlorphentermine S.A. in the treatment of obesity and the effect of weight loss on steroid excretion. *Br. med. J.* **2**, 453.

JAFFE, C. V. (1961). Obesity in general practice: a critical trial with a new appetite suppressant diethylpropion hydrochloride (Tenuate). *Med. Press,* **245**, 41.

KAY, L. L., PRINTZ, S., ROBINSON, M. S. & TENDLER, J. (1961). Benzphetamine in the management of obesity complicated by cardiovascular disease. *Sth West. Med.* 42.

KNEEBONE, G. M. (1966). Some aspects of the treatment of childhood obesity. *Med. J. Aust.* **2**, 751.

LAMBUSIER, P. (1967). Action of fenfluramine in the long term treatment of obesity. *Unpublished.*

LE RICHE, W. H. & CSIMA, A. (1967). A long-acting appetite suppressant drug studied for 24 weeks in both continuous and sequential administration. *Can. med. Ass. J.* **97**, 1016.

LORBER, J. (1966). Obesity in childhood. A controlled trial of anorectic drugs. *Archs Dis. Childh.* **41**, 309.

MUNRO, J. F., MacCUISH, A. C., WILSON, E. M. & DUNCAN, L. J. P. (1968). Comparison of continuous and intermittent anorectic therapy in obesity. *Br. med. J.* **1**, 352.

MUNRO, J. F., MacCUISH, A. G., MARSHALL, A., WILSON, E. M. & DUNCAN, L. J. P. (1969). Weight reducing affect of diguanides in obese non-diabetic women. *In Press.*

MUNRO, J. F., SEATON, D. A. & DUNCAN, L. J. P. (1966). Fenfluramine in the treatment of refractory obesity. *Br. med. J.* **2**, 624.

OSWALD, I., JONES, H. S. & MANNERHEIM, J. E. (1968). Effects of two slimming drugs on sleep. *Br. med. J.* **1**, 796.

PROCTOR, D. W. & STOWERS, J. M. (1967). Fatal lactic acidosis after an overdose of phenformin. *Br. med. J.* **4**, 216.

REE, M. J. (1962). Thyroid induced myxoedema. *Br. med. J.* **2**, 97.

REECE, C. H. (1963). The overweight patient in general practice. *Med. Wld, Lond.* **98**, 193.

RENDLE-SHORT, J. (1960). Obesity in childhood. A clinical trial of phenmetrazine. *Br. med. J.* **1**, 703.

ROGINSKY, M. S. & BARNETT, J. (1966). Double blind study of phenformin in weight control of obese non-diabetic subjects. *Am. J. clin. Nutr.* **19**, 223.

SEATON, D. A., DUNCAN, L. J. P., ROSE, K. & SCOTT, A. M. (1961). Diethylpropion in the treatment of refractory obesity. *Br. med. J.* **1**, 1009.

SEATON, D. A., ROSE, K. & DUNCAN, L. J. P. (1964). Sustained action chlorphentermine in the correction of refractory obesity. *Practitioner,* **193**, 698.

SENSENBACH, W. E. & HAYS, E. E. (1960). Iron exchange resins in the formulation of sustained release medication. *Am. J. med. Sci.* **240,** 474.

SILVERMAN, M. (1959). Subacute delirious state due to 'Preludin' addiction. *Br. med. J.* **1,** 697.

SILVERSTONE, J. T. (1968). Slimming and sleep. *Br. med. J.* **2,** 175.

SILVERSTONE, J. T. & SOLOMON, T. (1965). The long term management of obesity in general practice. *Br. J. clin. Pract.* **19,** 395.

SKIPPER, E. W., ORMEROD, T. P. & HASTE, A. R. (1968). Current therapeutics. 'Metformin.' *Practitioner,* **200,** 868.

SMITH, R. C. F. (1962). The long-term control of obesity with a sustained-release appetite suppressant. *Br. J. clin. Pract.* **16,** 415.

SPENCE, A. E. & MEDVEI, V. C. (1967). Fenfluramine in the treatment of obesity. *Br. J. clin. Pract.* **20,** 643.

TRAHERNE, J. B. (1965). Clinical trial of fenfluramine. *Practitioner,* **195,** 677.

WELSH, A. L. (1962). *Side Effects of Anti-Obesity Drugs.* Springfield, Illinois: Thomas.

WHITE, A. G., BECKETT, A. H. & BROOKES, L. G. (1967). Fenfluramine overdosage. *Br. med. J.* **1,** 740.

CHAPTER 8

The Treatment of Obesity by Exercise

OBESITY rarely occurs in heavy manual works or in energetic people with restless personalities and the role of exercise in the development of obesity has undoubtedly been underestimated in the past.

Mayer and his co-workers (1956) showed that calorie intake increases with activity within the zone of ' normal activity '. Below that range (the ' sedentary zone ') a decrease in activity is not followed by a decrease in food intake, but on the contrary by an increase. Body weight is also increased. These results were obtained by careful assessment of the amount of food bought by 213 mill workers in West Bengal but are likely to apply to all civilised communities (Fig. 4).

A criticism of this survey is that among the sedentary workers the stall-holders and supervisors were presumably better paid than the other workers and may have been able to afford more food. On the other hand the clerks, Group I, who lived on the premises and took no part in sporting activities were presumably in the same financial bracket as the three other groups of clerks who lived outside the works and commuted from three to six miles away daily, and it appears likely therefore that their calorie intake can be accounted for by the differing amounts of exercise taken.

Johnson, Burke & Mayer (1956) showed that inactivity was more important than over-eating when comparing 28 obese high school girls with 28 normal controls. The obese girls spent an average of four hours per week on active sport compared with the 11 hours per week of the controls.

Stefanik, Heald & Mayer (1959) assessed 14 obese boys and 14 normal controls at school and during summer camp and found that the obese boys preferred the less active exercises. Exercises involving running were preferred by three obese boys, but by eight of the controls.

BODY WEIGHT AND CALORIFIC INTAKE
AS A FUNCTION OF PHYSICAL ACTIVITY

(AFTER MAYER ET AL)

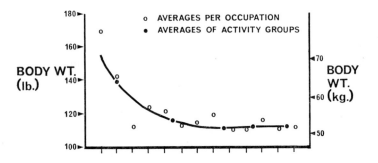

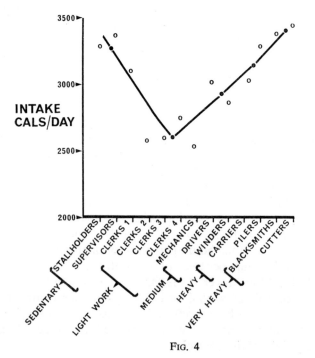

FIG. 4

Bloom & Eidex (1967) found on comparing seven obese housewives with six lean housewives, that the obese housewives on average spent an hour longer in bed than the lean and spent 15 per cent less time on their feet each day.

Dorris & Stunkard (1957) studied the amount of walking undertaken by 15 obese women and compared them with 15 normal controls. During one week the obese women walked 2·1 miles daily on average and the non-obese women 4·9 miles. The obese women had a different attitude to despondency and boredom from the controls, in that they tended towards a passive acceptance of the situation, whereas the controls took a more active attitude. Similar results were obtained in men by Chiroco & Stunkard (1960) who found that 25 obese men walked an average of only 3·7 miles per day compared with 6·0 miles per day for non-obese controls.

Stunkard & Peska (1962) found that 15 obese girls at a Girl Scout camp for two weeks walked an average of 7·2 miles a day, compared with 8·1 miles a day walked by 15 controls of normal weight, but a high level of activity was required of all the girls at camp which made it extremely difficult to show any differences in overall activity. As a result of this enforced exercise the obese girls maintained a steady weight on average while the controls gained an average of 0·8 kg. (1·8 lb.) each. This suggests that increased activity could lead to a loss of weight for the obese girls under normal circumstances.

McCarthy (1966) found no difference in the number of hours spent daily in different types of activity between 63 obese Trinidadian women and 26 normal controls. Both claimed to have approximately the same calorie intake. The explanation for this apparent discrepancy probably lies in the fact that obese women taking part in the same activity as non-obese are likely to expend less energy, as was proved in the case of girls by Bullen, Read & Mayer (1964). Motion pictures were taken of 109 obese girls aged 13 to 17 and 72 non-obese girls of the same age while they were participating in swimming, volley ball and tennis, which proved that the obese girls were much less active although they spent the same length of time on the sports.

Consumers' Association (1967) report that of their 3,000 members who admit to an overweight problem, half of them never take any exercise, and say that they are actually on the move for only an hour or less each day.

These findings as to the amount of exercise taken by obese people were confirmed in the author's practice. The amount of exercise was assessed by considering the answers to questions about the amount of energy expended in travelling to work, at work, and in sports and pastimes. The difference between the obese and the normal controls in exercise taken is significant at the 1 per cent level.

TABLE VIII

Amount of Exercise Taken in Author's Series

Amount of exercise	78 Obese	28 Obese controls	106 Obese Total	50 Normal controls
Below average	38 (49%)	18 (64%)	56 (53%)	8 (16%)
Above average	1 (1%)	0 (0%)	1 (1%)	6 (12%)

The role of exercise in weight reduction

For exercise to be effective in assisting weight reduction it must be taken daily and for adequate periods, as walking three miles in an hour merely utilises 300 calories in a person of average weight.

Three miles per day represents the average difference in miles walked per day between the obese women and the controls in Dorris & Stunkard's series, so that it should not be difficult to take this additional exercise. Alternatives to an hour's walking are three quarters of an hour's bicycling or half an hour of swimming or tennis. A further loss of weight varying for each individual must be added to the amounts shown in Table IX due to the increased metabolic rate resulting from exercise (p. 33). This additional weight loss may increase as the person loses weight because the metabolic rate will then increase more with exercise.

Many individuals, especially men, become obese on giving up regular exercise. The role of exercise in the treatment of obesity has been underestimated in the past because of theories as to the amount of exercise needed to 'work off' a certain weight of fat. However, if the exercise is taken daily and regularly, fat can be 'worked off' over a period of months to a considerable amount in the course of a year, as shown in Table IX.

TABLE IX

Additional Weight Loss from Exercise
(Modified from Keys)

One hour's walking daily (or $\frac{3}{4}$ hour's bicycling or $\frac{1}{4}$ hour's swimming or $\frac{1}{2}$ hour's tennis)

| Weight | | One month | | Two months | | Three months | |
kg.	(lb.)	kg.	(lb.)	kg.	(lb.)	kg.	(lb.)
59	(130)	1·0	(2·2)	2·0	(4·4)	2·9	(6·5)
66	(145)	1·1	(2·5)	2·2	(4·9)	3·3	(7·3)
73	(160)	1·3	(2·8)	2·5	(5·5)	3·7	(8·1)
79	(175)	1·4	(3·1)	2·6	(6·0)	4·0	(8·9)
86	(190)	1·5	(3·4)	2·9	(6·5)	4·3	(9·6)
102	(225)	1·8	(3·9)	3·5	(7·7)	5·1	(11·3)
113	(250)	2·0	(4·3)	3·9	(8·6)	5·7	(12·7)

After a period of weight reduction the rate of loss of weight from exercise diminishes as it is proportional to the original weight according to Keys, but this calculation takes no account of the ' bonus ' due to the temporary increase in metabolic rate resulting from the exercise.

An increase in the amount of regular exercise undertaken should be part of the weight reducing regime for every patient with no medical contra indication (see diet on p. 57).

With some obese patients you just can't win, however, as Buskirke (1967) has shown that when obese patients increase their amount of exercise and restrict their calorie intake, they compensate by sitting more quietly or lying more still!

Exercise machines

Stationary bicycles and ' rowing machines ' are obviously efficient aids to weight reduction if used regularly, but the various forms of vibratory machine, costing from £15 to £20 each, were tested by Consumers' Association (1967) and found to cause a loss of energy less than the amount of energy a person would normally use walking about slowly for the same time.

REFERENCES

BLOOM, W. L. & EIDEX, M. F. (1967). Inactivity as a major factor in adult obesity. *Metabolism*, **16**, 679.

BULLEN, B. A., READ, R. B. & MAYER, J. (1964). Physical activity of obese and non-obese adolescent girls appraised by motion picture sampling. *Am. J. clin. Nutr.* **14**, 211.

BUSKIRKE, E. R. (1967). Physical activity and cardiovascular health. *Can. med. Ass. J.* **96**, 785.

CHIROCO, A. M. & STUNKARD, A. J. (1960). Physical activity and human obesity. *New. Engl. J. Med.* **263**, 935.

CONSUMERS' ASSOCIATION (1967). *Which?*, 5th October.

DORRIS, P. J. & STUNKARD, A. J. (1957). Physiological activity performance and attitudes of a group of obese women. *Am. J. med. Sci.* **233**, 622.

JOHNSON, M. L., BURKE, B. S. & MAYER, J. (1956). Relative importance of inactivity and overeating on the energy balance of obese high school girls. *Am. J. clin. Nutr.* **4**, 37.

KEYS, A. & KEYS, Margaret (1960). *Eatwell & Staywell*. London: Hodder and Stoughton.

MAYER, J., ROY, P. & MITRA, K. P. (1956). Relation between caloric intake, body weight and physical work. *Am. J. clin. Nutr.* **4**, 169.

McCARTHY, M. G. (1966). Dietary and activity pattern of obese women in Trinidad. *J. Am. diet. Assn.* **48**, 37.

STEFANIK, P. A., HEALD, F. F. & MAYER, J. (1959). Caloric intake in relation to energy output of obese and non-obese adolescent boys. *Am. J. clin. Nutr.* **7**, 55.

STUNKARD, A. & PESTKA, J. (1962). The physical activity of obese girls. *Am. J. Dis. Childh.* **103**, 116.

CHAPTER 9

The Psychological Aspects of Obesity

PSYCHOLOGICAL ASPECTS IN AETIOLOGY

IN the early 1940's the concept of obesity as an expression of neurosis began to be ventilated and in 1946 Nicholson and his co-workers in a private obesity clinic at Duke Hospital, North Carolina, produced their classical study showing that the incidence of failure was high when a diet was the only form of treatment given and results were much better when psychotherapy was included.

In a series of 93 patients, a group of 38 patients treated by careful history taking, psychotherapy and explanation of calorie values, together with an assessment of a three-day food intake, were compared with 35 patients placed on a 800 calorie diet which was explained to them by a dietician; no effort at psychotherapy was attempted in the latter group. The family history of obesity was similar in the two groups. In the first group 26 out of 38 lost weight and in the second group only nine out of 35. A smaller group of 10 patients given amphetamine sulphate alone lost weight only to regain it and another group of 10 patients given thyroid hormone showed no appreciable weight loss.

The concept of the plump, rounded person being easy-going and happy requires some modification. Roundness gives an appearance of happiness and of course obese people as a rule move more slowly than the non-obese and therefore appear to be less tense. Nevertheless, some rounded people are only happy because they overeat.   .

The furthest that any of those who minimise the psychological aspects of obesity will go is to maintain that there are no more anxious or depressed people amongst the obese than in the general population.

In the U.S.A. Weinberg et al. (1960), applying six different psychological tests, found no difference between 18 obese men and 18 normal men and Friedman (1959) found no appreciable difference between 26 young obese college women, 26 normal controls and 26 underweight young women, except that the overweight and underweight women were less objective and more hypersensitive than the normal controls. He considered that this might be a result of the abnormal weight rather than the cause. Shipman & Plesset (1963) found no statistically significant differences between obese patients and normal controls when matched for similarity in age, sex, socio-economic and marital status. On the other hand, as a result of the Minnesota Multiphesic Personality Inventory (MMPI) and the Edwards Personal Preference Schedule (EPPS), Shipman & Heath (1966) found that 35 women, who had either volunteered for a research diet or applied for psychotherapeutic help, reported inner struggle but denied any social anxiety. They found three sub-groups: depressed dependant women, greedily demanding women and jolly and extroverted women; the last group tended to put on weight when married to a less vigorous man and the arrival of children meant immobilisation and frustration. Shipman & Heath point out that in a large group the sub-groups of depressed and extroverted women would tend to cancel each other out and give the group as a whole an average figure.

Moore and her colleagues (1962), in a very through investigation into the mental health of 334 obese men and women and 1,042 normal controls in New York City in 1962, found that the obese had more pathological scores in eight out of nine measures than the controls. The scores achieved statistical significance in immaturity, rigidity and suspiciousness. The obese persons were not a complete cross section of the obese population however, as they were those who had volunteered to attend obesity clinics.

Caufman & Pauley (1961) have presented perhaps the most conclusive evidence to date of the inter-relationship of obesity and psychological disorder by selecting 26 apparently emotionally normal obese patients (nine men and 17 women) out of a total of 200 obese patients and comparing the rate of weight loss with the results of psychological testing. The testing by the Cornell Medical Index showed that 13 of them (50 per cent) were probably emotionally abnormal (scores of 13 or more) compared with 20 per cent in the general population. All the patients were given prochlorperazine and dexamphetamine in sustained release form and a 1,000 calorie diet for an average period of seven weeks. Table X shows that the CMI scores rise steadily as dietary success decreases. After detailed history taking it was thought that three of the five diatetic failures probably needed psychiatric treatment.

TABLE X

Correlation of Weight Loss with C.M.I. Score
(After Caufman & Pauley)

Average Weight kg.	Weekly Loss (lb.)	% of Overweight	No. of Patients		C.M.I. Score Average	Range
1·4+	(3+)	12	3		6	4-10
0·9-1·4	(2-3)	9·9	9		9	0-29
0·4-0·9	(1-2)	7·8	9		8	1-19
0-0·4	(0-1)	2	2	3/5 needed treatment	17	1-35
0	0		3		26	13-36

Severely disturbed psychiatric patients are commonly overweight due to a combination of overeating and underactivity, stemming from psychological factors. Haward (1965) from Graylingwell Hospital, Chichester, points out that appetite reducing drugs are inadequate treatment as they do not reduce food intake in spite of reducing appetite.

Among patients in this country, Silverstone & Solomon (1965) in a London suburban general practice found that 41 out of 272 women between 20 and 60 who attended during a three month period were overweight. A weight reduction clinic was attended for a year by 31 of them and 23 completed the trial: 11 of the 31 were considered to be significantly neurotic by the C.M.I., which is not a significantly higher proportion than found in patients of London general practitioners. The *non-neurotic women lost more weight than the neurotic ones.*

7

Silverstone (1968) assessed 344 (77 per cent) of a one in five sample of adult patients in two London general practices; 85 (52 per cent) of the men were more than 15 per cent overweight and 102 (56 per cent) of the women. There was no significant difference in the incidence of neuroticism between the obese and the normal. Individuals were regarded as neurotic if they had 10 or more positive replies to the M.R. questions in the Cornell Medical Index.

More than 30 per cent overweight was found in 29 (18 per cent) of the men and 45 (25 per cent) of the women; 20 of the men and 30 of the women were matched with normal controls. None of the men was neurotic as shown by the C.M.I. but eight of the normal and 11 of the obese women could be so classified. *Food was very important to 11 of these obese women but only to six of the normal women, and 17 of the obese women admitted to eating more when anxious compared with seven of the controls.* Their anxiety would appear to have been expressed by overeating and consequent obesity instead of in other ways. These obese people represented a sample of all the overweight persons in the two practices, whereas in the previous survey the 31 of the original 42 obese patients who agreed to attend a weight reduction clinic were those who required advice and were thus self selective.

How can this conflicting evidence be reconciled? It appears to be generally accepted that at least as many obese people are anxious or depressed as in the general population, but many series have shown a greater incidence of psychological factors in the obese than in the normal. One reason for this is that they have consisted of people with a severe degree of obesity who have consulted their private practitioners, or have been referred to hospital clinics or to psychiatrists. This is only a small proportion of the total obese population and will necessarily include most of those with poor adjustment to their life situation. Reference to Table XI will show that *in the author's practice the obese controls are much nearer to the normal controls than they are to the obese patients.*

Another reason for divergence of results is in the varying social and racial groupings. For instance, obesity was six times more common in women of low social status in Manhattan than those of a high social class (Goldblatt *et al.*, 1965).

Obesity was also three times more common in women of Italian origin than in those of British descent. The social pressures which determine these vastly different incidences of obesity are bound to result in very different incidences of anxiety and depression which will lead to differing results of comparative psychological testing. *Obesity represents a syndrome rather than a disease entity.*

The author's results complement Silverstone & Soloman's findings. Psychiatric history taking was concerned with the patients' own opinion as to their happiness at the present time and in their childhood, their admission as to whether

TABLE XI

*Major Psychological Factors
in Author's Series*

*See Table XIV for overall results of series and page 120 for
criteria of success*

Factor	Obese Patients			Obese controls	Normal controls	All controls
	Dietary failures (or re-lapsed)	Dietary successes	All obese patients			
	51	27	78	28	50	78
Unhappy child-hood	13 (25%)	3 (11%)	16 (21%)	1 (4%)	4 (8%)	5 (6%)
Past history of nervous breakdown	11 (22%)	3 (11%)	14 (18%)	3 (11%)	2 (4%)	5 (6%)
Major worries now	16 (31%)	5 (19%)	21 (27%)	4 (14%)	8 (16%)	12 (15%)
Below average for happiness	6 (12%)	1 (4%)	7 (9%)	4 (14%)	3 (6%)	7 (9%)
Above average for happiness	15 (29%)	7 (26%)	22 (28%)	11 (39%)	15 (30%)	26 (33%)
Eats when depressed or nervy			24 (31%)	6 (21%)	9 (18%)	15 (19%)

they had ever sustained a nervous breakdown and as to whether they had anything worrying them in a major way at the present time. These general impressions cannot compare in thoroughness with the American reports based on detailed testing, but the results are nevertheless valid.

It can be seen from Table XI that a much larger proportion of obese patients had had an unhappy childhood or a nervous breakdown, while a larger proportion admitted to present worries. This tendency was increased in those who failed or relapsed and if this group is compared with the normal controls for these factors and that of present unhappiness in addition, the incidence is in each case at least twice that of the normal. There is also an increased tendency to eat when depressed or nervous.

In the author's series the treated obese comprised only about one-third of the total number of obese people in the practice.

The majority of obese people probably have no obvious psychological factors affecting their tendency to obesity. Many of them are people who eat under the minor stresses of every-day life instead of, or as well as smoking, drinking alcohol or tea or biting their nails. They do not bother to consult their doctors about the problem of overweight for a variety of reasons. Many of them are not distressed physically by their overweight and are not worried enough about their looks to consider the discipline of serious dieting. Many of them appear to overeat instead of getting depressed or neurotic. Some of them may indeed need to be large in body to compensate for feelings of inferiority as suggested by Bruch (1957b) and Yudkin (1959) and have a vested interest in remaining fat. Gluckman & Hirsh (1968) confirmed this need in four cases described in detail.

EATING AS A FORM OF COMPENSATION FOR LACK OF LOVE

In the author's experience of following up 177 cases of obesity and assessing 28 obese controls, those who need to eat as compensation for lack of love in their lives form a large and important group.

As long ago as 1931 Newburgh spoke of the ' individual who uses food as a comfort ' and more recently the concept of eating compensating an individual for lack of love has gained some measure of general acceptance. *These people are not necessarily anxious or depressed, as eating tends to relieve feelings of anxiety or depression before they have a chance to become organised. Eating therefore helps to keep them stable.*

Simon (1963) found that in the U.S. Air Force, overweight men were in fact far less depressed than normal controls and he concluded that obesity is a depressive equivalent. Only one out of 27 men were depressed for more than two weeks compared with 13 out of 50 normal controls. His findings are confirmed by the fact that the incidence of suicide is significantly less in the obese than in the general population (Table II).

The possibility of the existence of compensatory eating should therefore be considered when interviewing any new case of obesity. Three main groups of individuals seem to find compensation in eating, which may be the major or only pleasure in their lives.

1. Children lacking love from one or both parents (p. 165).
2. Single individuals or married couples with no children.
3. Unhappy individuals living in a state of stress and lack of general affection.

TABLE XII

Results of Dieting in Childless Individuals

Group	No Children	Children	Total
I and II (Success)	2	26	28
III and IV (Relapsed success)	6	18	24
V (Failure)	10	17	27
Total	18	61	79
Controls	20	59	79

Compensatory Eating in Childless Adults

Obesity commonly occurs as a result of eating to compensate for lack of children and this is confirmed in the author's series by comparing the numbers of childless individuals in the successful, relapsed and failed groups. The childless individuals in Table XII include single persons and those married, separated or widowed who have never had children. The difference between the successes (groups I and II) and the failures (group V) is statistically significant at the 5 per cent level.

Compensatory Eating in Adults under stress

Understanding this problem will be helped if individual cases are discussed, and many of the 27 failures in the author's five year follow-up group are of interest in this respect. Three of them were never seriously concerned about weight loss, although they would have liked to lose weight if it could be done without any trouble to themselves. When a diet was prescribed rather than the drugs they were hoping for they did not bother to return. Two were probably compensatory eaters. Two patients could be classed as relative successes in that both were ' only just ' obese; they had lost 6·5 kg. (1 stone) and 25 kg. (4 stones) respectively before entry into the trial and managed to maintain this previous weight loss.

All of the remaining 22 failures could be considered compensatory eaters. They can be divided into two main groups, the first being 12 fairly well adjusted people with something obviously lacking in their lives, who appear to accept their overeating as compensatory, and the second being 10 basically unhappy individuals with some constant stress. The well adjusted group include six childless married people and one single person. One openly admits that she eats because she cannot have children and another admits to obsessional eating. The group is completed by three grandmothers who have time on their hands, an unhappily married woman whose teenage children are beginning to grow away from her and the wife of an airline pilot who has to endure frequent separations from her husband. The group of 10 unhappy people are all women, most of whom have obvious major stress factors to contend with or suffer from depressive illness.

In the groups of relapsed successes it appears likely that 18 out of 24, including five of the six childless individuals, are compensatory eaters. Of the 28 obese controls it is possible that 12, including six of the seven childless individuals, are compensatory eaters. Of the 106 obese adults in the author's practice who were interviewed, therefore, a total of 54 individuals, 21 of whom were childless, appeared in some measure to derive pleasure from eating to compensate for lack of love in their lives. It is possible that up to half of the obese children in the practice eat to compensate for lack of parental affection.

OBESITY FOLLOWING EMOTIONAL SHOCKS

An abrupt onset of obesity following a severe emotional shock can occur occasionally and Bruch (1940) quotes two cases out of her series of 142 obese children. She also (1957b) mentions the case of the philosopher William Hume recorded in his *A Letter to a Physician* written in 1734 and other cases from her own experience. In this country in 1949 Shorvon & Richardson record six cases of obesity following emotional trauma. One of the author's patients showed similar features:

Mrs. J. S. was 23 when, in 1962, the younger of her two small boys, aged 15 months, was admitted to hospital with poliomyelitis involving his right leg and producing some paralysis. A month later she consulted the author because she had been worried and irritable since his admission and a tranquiliser was prescribed. She put on 9·5 kg. (21 lb.) in weight in the four months after her son was admitted to hospital. This represented 15 per cent of her weight before he was admitted.

Carbohydrate addiction. Many obese people have obsessions with eating and find it difficult to stop once they have started. They have eating ' binges ' similar to alcoholic binges and in some cases these urges to eat are uncontrollable by an effort of will. They commonly occur in the evening. A true metabolic craving for carbohydrate (p. 19) may be allied to the psychological craving, and it is reasonable to describe their condition as one of addiction to carbohydrates. Hamburgher (1951), describing 18 cases with known emotional causes for overeating, found that eight of them appeared to be addicted to carbohydrate. Bloom & Clarke (1964) give details of four cases which they call ' obese carboholics '. *Strict carbohydrate restriction is as essential in these cases as is abstention from* *alcohol to the alcoholic.* Similarly, moral support from the physician is essential for there to be any hope of prolonged remission, and short spells of anorectic drugs are needed in some cases. As with alcoholism one cannot speak of cure in these cases and with most of them there is a constant battle against the desire to eat carbohydrate food (Fig. 9). One of these patients on being asked ' you *do* love your food don't you? ' replied ' No I *worship* it '. Carbohydrate addicts lie about their intake of carbohydrate in the same way as alcoholics lie about their consumption of alcohol.

The fat person's attitude to obesity. Few obese people will talk freely to others about their feelings concerning their own overweight, but psychiatrists have given us a picture of the way some of them feel about themselves.

Bruch (1957b) states that Schilder, a neurologist, first mentioned the phrase ' *disturbance of the body image* ' in 1935 and that Bender applied the phrase to ' disturbed children ' in 1952. When these children drew a picture of a man, she regarded this as a self portrait and where this self portrait was bizarre she correlated this with the child having a schizoid personality. Bruch amplified this concept with regard to obese children and she feels that ' obese people live under the continuous pressure of a derogatory attitude in their environment towards their bodies '. Stunkard popularised the phrase ' disturbance of the body image '. He found that a number of obese patients feel that their bodies are loathsome and that others must view them with hostility and contempt. In most of his cases this attitude developed in adolescence, was associated with some emotional disturbance and a fear of derogatory remarks by their parents. Many of them fear that no one will want them as a sexual partner. Other young adolescents have similar feelings about disturbing physical characteristics such as a dark skin, the wearing of glasses, or braces for teeth. Stunkard & Birt (1967) contacted 10 of the 17 adults who were normal in weight out of Abraham & Nordsieck's follow-up into adulthood of 100 overweight children (1960). Three of these had suffered from disturbance of the body image and were much improved since weight reduction. Nevertheless, they were still preoccupied by their physical appearance and this fact makes it important to treat obesity early in childhood, to prevent the syndrome arising in adolescence. Bruch (1957b) calls these persons ' thin, fat people ', who may be made panicky by gaining less weight than an observer can detect. Stunkard feels that where disturbance of the body image occurs there is a specific indication for psychotherapy. These people are certainly all suffering from severe inferiority feelings which demand attention from their family doctor or from a psychiatrist.

CAN DIETING CAUSE DEPRESSION?

Stunkard (1957) reported that of 100 consecutive obese people requesting reducing diets at the Nutrition Clinic at the New York Hospital, 72 had dieted previously and 34 per cent of these complained of symptoms of weakness, nervousness, irritability and fatigue as a result of dieting. Of 25 people with obesity which was severe or difficult to manage, nine had severe emotional disorders, which he considered to be due to the dieting, and 20 were night eaters, who complained of insomnia or early morning waking.

These were all seriously overweight people however, who had been referred to a psychiatrist and Shipman & Plesset (1963) found that while 15 per cent of 151 patients from hospital and general practice were anxious or depressed at the beginning of treatment, approximately the same percentage were anxious or depressed at the end of treatment, and they consisted mainly of the same individuals.

The dangers of persisting with attempts at strict dieting without a full evaluation of a patient's background should be borne in mind, but in general practice depression is unlikely to be caused by dieting, unless there is a previous history of psychiatric illness, according to a trial involving 60 patients for 16 weeks reported by Silverstone & Lascelles (1966). None of the author's patients have appeared to become depressed following the free diet advised, as they have been free to discontinue the diet whenever they chose, and no pressure has been brought upon them to return for review except at the end of the survey.

As stated in relation to compensatory eating, many obese people have accepted overweight as an alternative to depression. As Hilda Bruch says (1957b) ' we must learn to recognise that for many people overeating and being fat is a balancing factor in their adjustment to life. Ineffective as it is, it represents the best form of adaptation that such people have been able to make '.

Successful dieting may in some cases lead to a diminution of anxiety and depression because whatever the original causes of tension or unhappiness in many cases the unpleasantness of being obese adds to them. Guilt due to overeating leads to further anxiety, and further overeating. Anxiety and depression were diminished by successful dieting in Shipman & Plesset's series. Successful dieting breaks the vicious circle and in many anxious or depressed patients, drugs and other aids to rapid weight reduction are fully justified to boost their morale (Chap. 13). It should, however, be borne in mind that these people are in danger of becoming addicts, and drugs must never be given for long periods without the most careful supervision (Case 5, p. 69).

A few patients are pathologically depressed as well as being obese and in these cases it is essential that the depression is treated as well as the obesity as the prognosis otherwise is very poor. Shipman & Plesset (1963) found that patients with scores of 15 or above on the depressive side of the A/D scale (p. 109) tended to diet for a long time, but unsuccessfully, and were likely to require psychological assessment. Fischer (1967) found that the persistence of significant depression made the actual loss of weight impossible. Of 20 obese women who had been fasted in hospital, 13 turned up for review 1 to $2\frac{1}{2}$ years later. The four of these who were classified as failures were those with the highest scores on the A/D scale. Fischer felt that this test showed inherited personality traits. These patients are usually sensitive people who worry excessively and have times when they feel useless.

Three out of the four patients in the author's practice who weighed over 130 kg. (20 stone) were typically jolly-looking, fat women, but two were severely depressed and required psychiatric help before weight loss could be achieved.

PROGNOSTIC FACTORS

As shown above, if a disturbance of the body image is present or there is a marked degree of depression, psychiatric help may be necessary if there is to be any real prospect of successful treatment. If there is a marked need to eat to compensate for lack of love, or from feelings of inferiority, successful weight reduction is unlikely to occur.

The author found that if the answers to two out of the four simple psychiatric questions patients were asked (p. 112, group 6) were unsatisfactory, failure or relapse was likely. In the obese series 15 out of the 18 patients with two of these factors were in the failed or relapsed group. Of the three successes, one had failed for about five years until an increase in dyspnoea gave her an incentive to lose weight (Fig. 8). One lost weight during a much wanted pregnancy and the third was probably in the early stages of diabetes when she achieved success in weight reduction after many years of failure. Only four of the obese controls had two of these factors and three of the remaining controls.

The author's four basic questions, therefore, help to give a guide to the outcome of treatment, and the Shipman A/D scale can give further help in assessing those who fail to lose weight or relapse easily.

In treating obese people with psychological problems it is important above all for the physician to understand and encourage his patients, and to avoid condemning them for not being able to lose weight, remembering the physician's role ' to cure sometimes, to relieve often, to comfort always '.

SHIPMAN ANXIETY DEPRESSION SCALE

This questionnaire consists of numbered statements. Read each statement and decide whether it is true as applied to you or false as applied to you. If it is *true* or *mostly true,* blacken the T to the left of the statement you are answering. If the statement is *not usually true* or is *not true at all,* blacken the F. Give your own opinion of yourself. Do not leave any blank spaces if you can avoid it.

T. F. 1. My daily life is full of things that keep me interested.

T. F. 2. I am easily awakened by noise.

T. F. 3. I believe I am no more nervous than others.

T. F. 4. At times I feel like smashing things.

T. F. 5. I work under a great deal of tension.

T. F. 6 My judgment is better than it ever was.

T. F. 7. I cannot keep my mind on one thing.

T. F. 8. I am a good mixer.

T. F. 9. I am more sensitive than most people.

T. F. 10. Everything is turning out just like the prophets in the Bible said it would.

T. F. 11. I frequently find myself worrying about something.

T. F. 12. Sometimes I keep on at a thing until others lose their patience with me.

T. F. 13. I am usually calm and not easily upset.

T. F. 14. I sometimes tease animals.

T. F. 15. I am happy most of the time.

T. F. 16. I usually feel that life is worthwhile.

T. F. 17. I have periods of such great restlessness that I cannot sit long in a chair.

T. F. 18. I go to church almost every week.

T. F. 19. I have sometimes felt that difficulties were piling up so high that I could not overcome them.

T. F. 20. I believe in the second coming of Christ.

T. F. 21. I certainly feel useless at times.

T. F. 22. I do not worry about catching disease.

T. F. 23. I find it hard to keep my mind on a task or job.

T. F. 24. Criticism or scolding hurts me terribly.

T. F. 25. I am not usually self-conscious.

T. F. 26. I certainly feel useless at times.

T. F. 27. I am inclined to take things hard.

T. F. 28. At times I feel like picking a fist fight with someone.

T. F. 29. I am a high strung person.

T. F. 30. Sometimes, when embarrassed, I break out into a sweat which annoys me greatly.

T. F. 31. Life is a strain for me much of the time.

T. F. 32. I enjoy many different kinds of play and recreation.

T. F. 33. At times I think I am no good at all.

T. F. 34. I like to flirt.

T. F. 35. I am certainly lacking in self-confidence.

T. F. 36. I brood a great deal.

T. F. 37. Sometimes I feel I am about to go to pieces.

T. F. 38. I sweat very easily even on cool days.

T. F. 39. I shrink from facing a crisis or difficulty.

T. F. 40. When I leave home I do not worry about whether the door is locked and the windows closed.

T. F. 41. I do not blame a person for taking advantage of someone who lays himself open to it.

T. F. 42. At times I am full of energy.

T. F. 43. Once in a while I laugh at a dirty joke.

T. F. 44. I feel anxiety about something or someone almost all the time.

The anxiety score in the above scale is the total of the following answers:

3.F	13.F	25.F	35.T
5.T	17.T	27.T	37.T
7.T	19.T	29.T	39.T
9.T	21.T	31.T	44.T
11.T	23.T	33.T	

The depressive score is the total of the following:

1.F	10.F	20.F	30.F	40.F
2.T	12.F	22.F	32.F	41.F
4.F	14.F	24.T	34.F	42.F
6.F	16.F	26.T	36.T	43.F
8.F	18.F	28.F	38.F	

Normal statistics based on 113 general population adults are:

Anxiety: Mean 6·8   Standard Deviation 4·2
Depression: Mean 10·5   Standard Deviation 2·9.

The validity and reliability of the above scale was assessed by Shipman (1963).

REFERENCES

ABRAHAM, A. & NORDSIECK, M. (1960). Relationship of excess weight in children and adults. *Publ. Hlth. Rep., Wash.* **75**, 263.

BLOOM, W. L. & CLARKE, M. B. (1964). The obese carboholic. *J. Obesity,* **1**, 10.

BRUCH, H. (1940). Physiologic and psychologic aspects of the food intake of obese children. *Am. J. Dis. Childh.* **59**, 739.

BRUCH, H. (1957a). Psychiatric aspects of obesity. *Metabolism,* **6**, 461.

BRUCH, H. (1957b). *The Importance of Overweight.* New York: Norton.

CAUFMAN, W. J. & PAULEY, W. G. (1961). Obesity and emotional status. *Penn. med. J.* **64**, 505.

FISCHER, N. (1967). Obesity, affect and therapeutic starvation. *Archs gen. Psychiat.* **17**, 227.

FRIEDMAN, J. (1959). Weight problems and psychological factors. *J. consult. Psychol.* **23**, 524.

GLUCKMAN, M. L. & HIRSCH, J. (1968). The response of obese patients to weight reduction; a clinical evaluation of behaviour. *Psychosom. Med.* **30**, 1.

GOLDBLATT, P. B., MOORE, M. E. & STUNKARD, A. J. (1965). Social factors in obesity. *J. Am. med. Ass.* **192**, 1039.

HAMBURGHER, W. W. (1951). Emotional aspects of obesity. *Med. Clins N. Am.* **35**, 483.

HAWARD, L. R. C. (1965). The inadequacy of anorexogenic drugs in the treatment of obese psychiatric patients. *Psychiatria Neurol.* **149**, 129.

MOORE, M. E., STUNKARD, A. J. & SROLL, L. (1962). Obesity social class and mental illness. *J. Am. med. Ass.* **181**, 962.

NEWBURGH, L. H. (1931). The cause of obesity. *J. Am. med. Ass.* **97**, 1659.

NICHOLSON, W. J. (1946). Emotional factors in obesity. *Am. J. med. Sci.* **211**, 443.

SHIPMAN, W. G. & HEATH, H. A. (1966). Personality subgroups among obese women. *Unpublished.*

SHIPMAN, W. G. (1963). A one-page scale of anxiety and depression. *Psychiat. Res. Rep.* **13,** 289.

SHIPMAN, W. G. & PLESSET, M. R. (1963). Anxiety and depression in obese dieters. *Archs gen. Psychiat.* **8,** 530.

SHORVON, H. J. & RICHARDSON, J. S. (1949). Depression in obese dieters. *Br. med. J.* **2,** 951.

SILVERSTONE, J. T. & LASCELLES, B. D. (1966). Dieting and depression. *Br. J. Psychiat.* **112,** 513.

SILVERSTONE, J. T. & SOLOMON, T. (1965). Psychiatric and somatic factors in the treatment of obesity. *J. Psychosom. Res.* **9,** 249.

SILVERSTONE, J. T. (1968). Psychosocial aspects of obesity. *Proc. R. Soc. Med.* **61,** 371.

SIMON, R. I. (1963) Obesity as a depressive equivalent. *J. Am. med. Ass.* **183,** 208.

STUNKARD, A. J. (1957). The dieting depression. *Am. J. med. Sci.* **23,** 77.

STUNKARD, A. & BIRT, V. (1967). Obesity and the Body Image. II. Age of onset of disturbance in the body image. *Am. J. Psychiat.* **123,** 1443.

STUNKARD, A. & MENDELSON, N. (1961). Disturbances in body images of some obese persons. *J. Am. Diet. Assoc.* **38,** 328.

WEINBERG, N., MENDELSON, M. & STUNKARD, A. (1960). A failure to find distinctive psychological features in a group of obese men. *Am. J. Psychiat.* **117,** 1035.

WERKMAN, S. L. & GREENBERG, E. S. (1967). Personality and interest patterns in obese adolescent girls. *Psychosom. Med.* **29,** 72.

YUDKIN, J. (1959). The causes and cure of obesity. *Lancet,* **2,** 1135.

CHAPTER 10

The Rational Treatment of Obesity

AS the preceding chapters have shown, simple obesity is a very individual complaint and for treatment to be rational, it must be tailored to each individual's problems after a careful assessment of the factors bearing on his tendency to eat more than his body needs.

The author has devised a questionnaire which includes most of the questions for which an answer is necessary in order to obtain a reasonable idea as to the best line of treatment for each particular case. This questionnaire can be given to the patient to complete while he is waiting to see the doctor, which saves time as well as ensuring that no essential points are missed whilst taking the history.

After history taking is completed the patient should be weighed and the height measured. The weight should be recorded to the nearest quarter-kilogram or half-pound in normal indoor clothes without shoes, on an accurate weighing machine.

The amount of clinical obesity is assessed if necessary (p. 2) and after the build has been noted, the best weight is estimated from the Tables (Appendix I). The author takes the upper limit of the weight given as the patient's best weight, to give him the benefit of the doubt unless it is known that he weighed less than this while in good health in his twenties. The blood pressure is recorded and the urine tested; the heart and lungs are examined if the blood pressure is raised or if dyspnoea is a complaint.

The physician is now in a position to advise the patient as to the best means of losing excessive weight.

A SCHEME FOR ASSESSING THE OVERWEIGHT PERSON

Please answer the following questions as accurately and completely as you can, as it will help your doctor to give you the best advice about tackling your problem.

1. Why do you want to lose weight? ....
   (a) Are you upset about the way you look?   Yes/No
   (b) Do you get breathless when you walk up hills? Yes/No
   (c) Does your overweight bother you in any other
       way?   Yes/No

2. When did you start to be overweight?   ....
   Why do you think you put on extra weight?   ....
   What was your weight in your early twenties? ....
   Have you dieted at any time?   Yes/No

3. Are any of your family overweight? If so state
   which:
       Father or mother.
       Grandparents.
       Uncles and aunts.
       Brothers and sisters.
       Children.

4. Do any of your family suffer from diabetes? If
   so state which.   ....

5. How many meals do you eat in a day?   ....
   How often do you have a really good ' gorge '? ....
   Do you eat between meals?   Yes/No
   How much alcohol do you take daily?   ....
   Do you prefer sweet things or savoury?   ....
   Do you eat when you are worried?   Yes/No
   Do you eat when you are unhappy?   Yes/No

6. Are you happy now?   Average. Above average. Below
       average.
   Did you have a happy childhood?   Yes/No
   Have you ever had a nervous breakdown?   Yes/No
   Have you any important worries at the moment? Yes/No

7. *Exercise.*
   How do you travel to work?   ....
   What sort of work do you do?   ....
   Do you use much energy in your work?   ....
   How many miles do you walk daily?   ....
   Do you have any active hobbies or recreations? ....

MEDICAL ASSESSMENT

1. Build: average, broad or narrow.
2. Weight: with shoes .... without shoes ....
3. Best weight ....
4. Number of pounds overweight ....
5. Clinical examination:

    (a) Excessive subcutaneous adipose tissue . + . + + .
                                                 + + +

    (b) Blood pressure
    (c) Heart and lungs
    (d) Urine

Each patient will need advice about diet which in most cases should be one of the free diets low in carbohydrates. Most patients will require to be encouraged to take more exercise, and in many cases their life situation should be surveyed to find out whether they display a tendency to com‑pensatory eating. A few patients who are only moderately overweight can be encouraged to accept their obesity as a reasonable adjustment to a difficult life situation. In some others to whom loss of weight is important for their self‑esteem and in whom the pressure to eat is great, it is reason‑able to commence treatment with drugs immediately. Almost all patients will be helped by the personal interest which the physician displays in their problem, his appreciation of their metabolic difficulties and of the pressures on them to eat more than they know is good for them. Most people should be seen again after an interval not exceeding two weeks. This period of time is selected as one for which most people can keep to a diet. Patients are told that if they keep strictly to the diet for two weeks, their new habit of eating will be becoming established, they will have lost an appreciable amount of weight and they will then be encouraged to carry on. As a general rule those who ask for reducing tablets are told that they can have them for a short period later on if they wish, to help them adhere to the diet but that if they rely on drugs initially their weight will increase immediately they leave off the drugs, unless they have already begun to alter their eating habits.

Those who attend for follow-up can be seen at fortnightly

intervals or more frequently on several further occasions, and then at approximately monthly intervals until the desired weight loss has been achieved, or until the curve of their weight loss has flattened out and it is obvious that they have not the motivation to carry on. Those who reach or approach their ' best weight ' can be advised to modify their diet by taking a few items which they had particularly missed while they were dieting strictly, but they should be told that they will always have to keep a check on their weight and should attend again for consultation if they ever had difficulty in keeping their weight down. An exception can be made in patients who have materially increased the amount of exercise they take.

At first sight it might appear that the suggestion that patients should lose between 2 and 7 kg. (5 and 15 lb.) per month on a free diet is unreasonable, but these figures are based on the author's early experience in the use of his modification of Marriott's diet and are confirmed by his own results. Of the patients in his early series who achieved initial success, 19 lost an average of 2·7 kg. (6 lb.) with a range of 1 to 4 kg. (2 to 9 lb.) in two weeks, and nine, who returned after exactly four weeks on the diet, lost an average of 4·5 kg. (9·5 lb.) with a range of 2·25 to 6·4 kg. (5 to 14 lb.).

FAILURE TO ACHIEVE WEIGHT LOSS

Those who do not lose weight at the end of two weeks or who have difficulty in maintaining their weight loss are questioned about the details of their dieting. It is often helpful for patients to write out in detail all the food they have consumed during a three-day period. In most cases there will be some obvious departures from the diet which they had been given. One of the author's patients took several spoonfuls of honey each night before retiring, to a total of one pound per week, her excuse being that honey was not specifically mentioned as forbidden on the diet sheet. In some cases the diet may require modification in one or more directions. The elimination of fruit and vegetables of a high calorie value per ounce from the diet may be necessary; these include bananas, peas, broad beans and corn. (Appendix II).

In those who have real difficulty in losing weight or main-taining weight loss, a further search should be made for a reason for compensatory eating. The Shipman A/D Scale (p. 107) will help in assessing the importance of psychological factors, and deciding whether psychiatric help is needed.

' *Successful management (of obesity) when it does occur, is the result of a knowledgeable sympathetic physician having the time and the interest to meet repeatedly with a patient who has at least a modicum of insight into the condition and a considerable motivation to reverse it* '. (Professor C. H. Hollen-berg of McGill University.)

CHAPTER 11

The Long-term Results of Treatment

A REVIEW of the literature reveals the paucity of long-term follow-ups in either the hospital or family doctor field. Many of the so-called 'long-term' follow-ups have been for periods of less than a year (one was for 18 weeks only) and most of these omit to record the failure rate. Stunkard & McLaren-Hume (1959) could find only eight reports which included all the original patients in their follow-ups. In their own series of 100 consecutive patients at the Nutrition Clinic of the New York Hospital only two of the patients who had lost 20 lb. or more had maintained their loss at the end of two years. Perhaps the most successful long-term follow-up of this era was by McCann & Trulson (1955) who followed up all except two of 180 patients who were alive and in the district at the end of three years. Regarding these two patients as failures, 35 (23 per cent) out of 149 patients had lost at least 30 per cent of their excess weight, and 5 (3 per cent) were within the normal range.

Glennon (1966) reviewed the literature since 1958 and could not find a successful long-term study. His series of obese subjects at least 50 per cent above their ideal weight, were all admitted to hospital where they lost an average of 6·8 kg. (15 lb.) in 12 days on a 1,000 calorie diet. Two years later they had regained 3·2 kg. (7 lb.) of this on average, but 23 of the 215 (10 per cent) had maintained 9·5 kg. (20 lb.) weight loss after one year and 14 (6 per cent of the original series) after two years. Only one subject attained the ideal weight.

From a wide experience in hospital and office practice, Strang (1964) estimates that only one in four patient will carry on a weight-reducing programme for one year and that only half of these, i.e. *one-eighth* of the total will maintain a truly long-term weight control.

Feinstein (1961) estimates that in the United States, of patients who achieve a significant weight loss only 1 to 2 per cent maintain this loss for five years. Glomset (1957) states that less than 10 per cent of patients achieve the desired weight loss, and 75 per cent of these have regained weight by the end of two years, therefore after two years he estimates that only $2\frac{1}{2}$ per cent maintain their weight loss. In Finland, Kotilainen (1963) found that even amongst voluntary weight losers only 7·5 per cent maintained the original weight loss for over three years. The volunteers were those who answered newspaper advertisements concerning the treatment of obesity.

A special group of volunteers in New York succeeded far better than any other group in the literature (Christakis *et al.*, 1966). The Anti-coronary Club of New York consisted of men aged between 40 and 59 at entry. After four years on a 1,600 calorie low-fat diet 134 (71·7 per cent) of the 187 obese at entry had become non-obese (less than 15 per cent above optimum weight) while only 20 (13·4 per cent) out of 149 controls, recruited from men who had voluntarily appeared for examination at cancer detection clinics, became non-obese. In spite of the fact that a loss of only a small amount may be necessary to cross the dividing line between obesity and ' normality ' this is still a remarkable result. Fear of coronary artery disease and frequent free health checks may have had a bearing on the type of person who volunteered, and weekly consultations gave them an extra incentive to keep to the diet (p. 53).

The best actual five-year follow-up is quoted by Dublin (1953) who states that 20 years previously Fellows had found that of 300 employees of the Metropolitan Life Insurance Company, 193 were available for follow-up five years later and 21 per cent of these, i.e. 13 per cent of the original 300, had maintained *some* weight loss. Social and economic conditions have changed so much over the last 20 or 30 years that this series is not strictly comparable with more recent ones.

In general practice, Lord (1966) followed up 40 cases for over two years at an overweight clinic in a cottage hospital assisted by a health visitor, who advised the patients concerning food values and diets. Eight patients were successful in losing half or more of their surplus weight and seven were partially successful initially, but there was only one success and one partial success from among 10 patients who still continued to attend the clinic at the end of two years (5 per cent of the original 40). Solomon (Silverstone & Solomon, 1965) started a special clinic for women more than 12·75 kg. (2 stones) above average weight who attended his surgery during a three-month period. Of 41 patients in this category, 31 accepted the offer of treatment and a double blind trial was undertaken comparing the use of diethylpropion and a placebo. All patients were also given a low carbohydrate diet. Eight of those on the drug and five on the placebo lost 6·4 kg. (1 stone) or more in the course of a year, which is just over one-third of these 31 patients.

Summary of Results from the Literature

It can be seen that, apart from the special case of the New York Anti-coronary Club, somewhere between 10 and 40 per cent of patients may have lost weight by the end of the first year, but the proportion of successes diminishes with the length of follow-up and by the end of five years the literature suggests that only between 1 and 13 per cent of patients have maintained some weight loss.

RESULTS IN THE AUTHOR'S PRACTICE

In the author's practice results were better than any of the above except for the New York Anti-coronary Club.

The practice. This is in a suburban area and has been established for over 100 years. There is a high proportion of office workers and artisans in the practice population, but a complete cross-section of the community is included, from directors to dustmen. The practice population at the beginning of the trial numbered about 2,000 and 2¾ years later, at the end of the period of entry into the trial, about 2,400. The practice at this time therefore represented a fairly typical English general practice.

The trial. All patients who were put on a diet for medical reasons were included in the trial, together with those who asked for advice regarding obesity. None of these patients was less than 10 per cent over his or her ' best ' weight. Those women who were given dietetic advice during the course of pregnancy were excluded from the trial. The total number of patients included was 100, of whom seven had died and eight had left the district five years later. Of the remaining 85 patients, six were children. A total of 79 adults, comprising nine men and 70 women, were therefore the subject of the survey. All were interviewed when they had been in the trial for between five and seven and three-quarter years, with the exception of one man who died after five years, but before he was due for interview.

The selection of a control group. A list in alphabetical order is kept for each year during which patients in the practice were born. Males and females are listed separately. These lists are known as the alphabetical age/sex register of the practice. At any time, therefore, the total number of each sex born in a given year may be known. The person whose name appeared in the register below that of each patient in the trial was selected as the normal control, providing that he or she had been in the practice at the end of the period of entry into the trial. Of the 78 controls, 14 were either already in the survey or had sought advice concerning obesity during the five years and so the next names on the age/sex register were substituted. The normal control patients were each sent a letter asking them to help in the research and inviting them to be seen by appointment.

A control series matched by age and sex should be comparable in every way with the group and, in this case, this was confirmed by comparing the heights of the women in the two series. The range was almost identical and the average height in each group was 5 ft. 2½ in. The group of nine men was too small for analysis.

Comparisons with the control group. Of the final 78 ' normal ' controls a total of 28 were at least 10 per cent overweight and another 27 were less than 10 per cent overweight, a mere 23 being in the normal range or below it. In some comparisons between obese patients and controls therefore, it seemed wise to compare the 106 obese patients, i.e. 78 in the series plus 28 obese controls, with the controls of normal weight or less than 10 per cent overweight, totalling 50.

The majority of the series (64 out of 79) consisted of women between 30 and 69 years of age. All were at least 10 per cent overweight, 55 were 20 per cent overweight and six were 50 per cent overweight.

TABLE XIII

Age at Onset of Survey

Age Group	Men	Women	Total
20 - 29		2	2
30 - 39	2	13	15
40 - 49	2	18	20
50 - 59	2	19	21
60 - 69	1	14	15
70 and over	2	4	6
Total	9	70	79

TABLE XIV

Overall Results

Group	No. of Patients	Average Loss	Result
I. Successful	14	8·1 kg. (18 lb.)	28 Successes (35·4%)
II. Partly successful	14		
III. Successful but relapsed	13	7·7 kg. (17 lb.) Initially	24 Relapses (30·4%)
IV. Partly successful but relapsed	11		
V. Failures	27	−3·2 kg. (−7 lb.)	27 Failures (34·2%)

Criteria of Success. Success in weight reduction should be related to the individual's initial weight or to the amount that he or she is overweight. In the author's survey the criterion of success selected was a loss at the end of survey period of at least 10 per cent of the initial weight. As a proportion of the total amount overweight this varied from 25 per cent to 100 per cent although usually in the range of 40 to 60 per cent so that many of the ' successes ' remained considerably over-weight. The loss of 5 per cent of the original weight (usually 20 to 40 per cent of excess weight) was regarded as ' partial success '. See page 126 for other criteria of success.

OVERALL RESULTS

It will be seen from Table XIV that by adopting these criteria one-third of the patients were successful or partly successful, one-third relapsed after having been successful or partly successful and the remaining one-third failed completely.

Since the main survey ended, a further 41 patients have been assessed after five years with a similar pattern of success, except for a proportionate increase in patients in group II.

DIFFERING PATTERNS OF SUCCESSFUL WEIGHT LOSS

The successful group I included 14 individuals who reacted in several different ways to dieting:

1. Six people lost considerable weight when they dieted initially, increased their weight slightly after the period of strict dieting ended and maintained a weight slightly above their lowest weight for many years, e.g. Mrs. E. A. Figure 5.

2. Three others lost considerable weight initially and continued to lose a little more over several years, e.g. Mr. E. G. Figure 6.

3. One lost weight in three successive steps, the first two by dieting alone and the third with the help of diethylpropion, e.g. Mrs. E. T. Figure 7.

4. Three lost no weight or put weight on for several years and then suddenly lost a considerable amount of weight. Two developed physical symptoms or signs, while the other increased her exercise considerably after the death of her husband, e.g. Mrs. A. H. Figure 8.

5. The remaining patient is in a class of her own on several counts. She is the only 127 kg. (20 stone) patient in the Group, her weight loss commenced for no obvious reason and continued throughout a much wanted pregnancy; she was 13·6 kg. (30 lb.) lighter at her post-natal than she was when three months pregnant. She later developed diabetes which probably accounted for the unexpected weight loss.

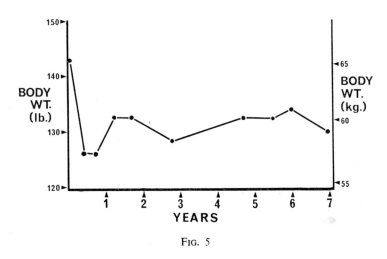

Fig. 5

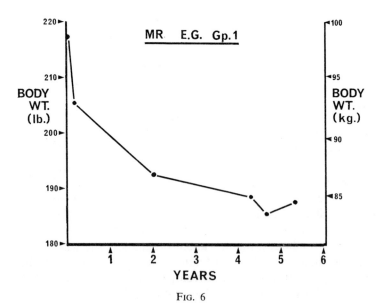

Fig. 6

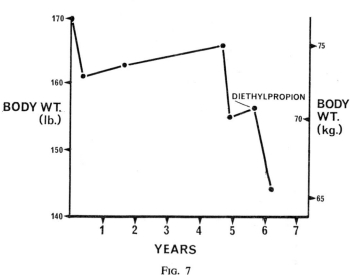

Fig. 7

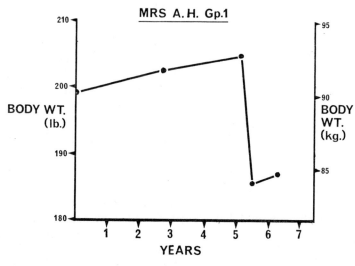

Fig. 8

Of the partly successful group II, of 14 individuals, the following results were recorded:

1. Four were successful on a minor scale and had similar patterns to those in group I. One like Figure 5, two like Figure 6 and one like Figure 8. This patient dieted successfully when her hiatus hernia became symptomatic.

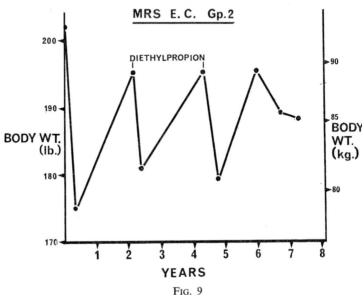

Fig. 9

2. Relapses occurred at some time in 10 patients.
   (a) Six, after an initial weight loss, had a series of partial relapses, e.g. Mrs. E. C. Figure 9.
   (b) Two, after initial success, had late relapse after four and six years respectively of successful dieting, e.g. Mrs. H. H. Figure 10.
   (c) Two had each a complete relapse with partial success later.

Many of the relapses in groups III and IV came fairly soon after the initial weight loss had occurred, but six of them were after two or three years, so that in a two-year follow-up most of these would have been classified as successes. Five individuals in these two groups had three or four successful dieting spells during the five to eight years of the survey. Two of these five would have been classified in groups I or II after

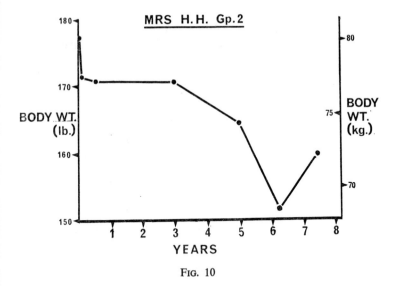

five or six years if the time of the end of the survey happened to coincide with the period following a spell of successful dieting.

Of the failures in group V three would have been successes and one a partial success had the entry into the trial been at a different time, as each of them put on considerable weight after entry and later lost an average of nearly 9·1 kg. (20 lb.) each after dieting, two for medical reasons.

It can be seen from the above details that a total of only 14 of the series were initially successful and maintained their weight loss without relapse, while two of the failures had previously lost weight successfully and had maintained their weight loss while still being overweight. *Thus a total of only 16 (21 per cent) of the original series were successful immediately and maintained their success over five years, or maintained a previously successful weight loss.* During the 2½ years since the main survey ended, five of the patients have died, six have left the district and two lost weight on developing diabetes, leaving 66 of the original 79 cases. Of these, 16 changed their groups, so that even a five-year survey does not give an adequate picture of what happens to obese people in the long term (Table XV).

TABLE XV

Comparison of 5-Year Survey with 7½-Year Survey

Group	5 Years (average 6½ years) No. of Patients	7½ Year (average 9 years) No. of Patients
I. Successful	10 ⎫	8 ⎫
II. Partly success-ful	11 ⎭ 21 Successes	18 ⎭ 26 Successes
III. Successful but relapsed	8 ⎫	7 ⎫
IV. Partly success-ful but relapsed	11 ⎭ 19 Relapses	8 ⎭ 15 Relapses
V. Failures	26 Failures	25 Failures
Total	66	66

Six patients had moved into a lower group, and 10 patients had moved into a higher group, resulting in a higher proportion of successes as compared to relapses. All the failures remained in the same group with one exception, but most of the other patients showed evidence of running an unstable course.

Success by Other Criteria

20 lb. weight loss. Many series quote a weight loss of 20 lb. (which is equal to approximately 9 kg.) as successful. In this series, 25 out of 94 patients (26 per cent) lost more than this amount at some time and nine out of 79 (11 per cent) maintained this loss for at least five years and an average of 6½ years.

Achieving normal weight. Adopting the stricter criterion of a patient losing enough weight to bring him or her within 10 per cent of his desirable weight (upper limit), i.e. no longer ' obese ', only 6 patients achieved this, of whom two were men. This represents a mere 7·7 per cent of the whole and only 5·7 per cent of the women.

Table XVI
Summary of Group Averages

Group	Male	Female	Total	Av. age	Wt. range at entry	Av. wt.	Average overweight	Av. wt. at end	Weight loss Av.	Weight loss % of orig.	Weight loss % of overwt.	Medical Reason	Drugs
I	3	11	14	54	128-273	180	46	157	23	12	52	9	7
II	1	13	14	53	150-220	177	45	165	12	7	27	7	9
III	1	12	13	55	128-212	167	35	165	2 / **21**	1 / **12**	6 / **60**	7	7
IV	1	10	11	41	148-198	163	33	165	+2 / **12**	**8**	**37**	3	7
V	3	24	27 / **15**	47	132-218	165	35	166	+1 / **12**	**7**	**34**	6	19
I & II	4	24	28	53	128-273	179	46	161	18	10	39	16	16
III & IV	2	22	24	48	128-212	165	34	165	0 / **17**	**10**	**50**	10	14

* Bold figures = weight lost at some time.

Some weight loss. Adopting the very much less strict criterion of ' some weight loss ' and excluding a loss of less than 1·3 kg. (3 lb), as was done by Dublin (1953), 43 out of 79 (54 per cent) had lost ' some weight' after five years, and 12 (15 per cent) were stationary.

An even less satisfactory criterion adopted by some authorities is the loss of 10 per cent of the excess weight. This may amount to as little as 1 or $1\frac{1}{2}$ kg. (2 or 3 lb.) in some cases.

COMPARISONS BETWEEN SERIES FROM GENERAL PRACTICE AND HOSPITAL

A comparison between a general practice series and a hospital series must take into account the type of case included in the hospital series. A series of cases of obesity *per se* consists of the more refractory cases referred from general practice and the bias is in favour of the general practice series. On the other hand, if the hospital series consists of obesity occurring in a medical clinic, all will have a medical reason for losing weight and there will be a bias in favour of the hospital series as obese patients are more likely to keep to a diet if there is an immediate medical benefit resulting from weight loss.

In this series 32 of the patients had a medical reason for losing weight, mainly on account of dyspnoea on exertion (17 patients), pain from osteo-arthritis of the weight bearing joints (10 patients) and symptoms from hiatus hernia (two patients). Of these 16 (50 per cent) were successful or partly successful. In addition five others were successful until their medical conditions had resolved; if these are included the successes total 21 out of 32 (65 per cent). These successes compare with 12 out of 47 (26 per cent) of those without a medical reason. This difference is significant at the 5 per cent level.

REFERENCES

CHRISTAKIS, G., RINZLER, S. H., ARCHER, H. & KRAUS, A. (1966). Effect of the anti-coronary club program on coronary heart disease risk-factor status. *J. Am. med. Ass.* **198,** 597.

DUBLIN, L. I. (1953). Benefits of reducing. *Am. J. Publ. Hlth,* **43,** 995.

FEINSTEIN, A. R. (1961). The problem of treatment in obesity. G.P. 23, 5:83.

GLENNON, J. A. (1966). Weight reduction—an enigma. *Archs intern. Med.* **118,** 1.

GLOMSET, D. A. (1957). Group therapy for obesity. *J. Iowa St. med. Soc.* **47,** 496.

KOTILAINEN, M. (1963). Group therapy for obesity; a study of results obtained at weight reducing courses in Finland. *Ann. Med. Intern. Fen.* **52,** 155.

LORD, W. J. H. (1966). Health education about obesity. The results of a two-year follow-up. *J. Coll. gen. Practnrs,* **11,** 285.

McCANN, M. & TRULSON, M. F. (1955). Long term effects of weight reducing programs. *J. Am. diet. Ass.* **31,** 1108.

SILVERSTONE, J. T. & SOLOMON, T. (1965). The long-term management of obesity in general practice. *Br. J. clin. Pract.* **19,** 395.

STRANG, J. M. (1964). In *Diseases of Metabolism.* Ed. Duncan, G. G. 5th ed. Philadelphia: Saunders.

STUNKARD, A. J. & McLAREN-HUME, M. (1959). The results of treatment for obesity. *Archs intern. Med.* **103,** 79.

CHAPTER 12

Prognosis

IT will be shown in Chapter 15 that the obese child is much more likely to grow into an obese adult than one of normal weight. It is therefore natural to suppose that *adults who have been obese from childhood are less likely to achieve success with diets than those who have become obese while adult,* and this has been shown to be the case in a survey of 2,593 clinic patients in New York City (Christakis, 1967). Amongst adults the age at which treatment for obesity is commenced does not necessarily make any difference. Women over 40 were more successful in the New York survey than younger women, but in the author's practice the average ages of the successful groups were not significantly different from the failures (Table XVI).

What are the other factors of help to the physician in deciding how difficult his patient is likely to find the problem of losing weight, and more important, of maintaining his weight loss? *Gross obesity is always a more difficult problem than an obesity of moderate degree.* The New York survey showed this, as have several others including Glennon's (1966). In a general practice gross obesity is not often encountered. If 127 kg. (20 stone) is taken as the dividing line, all those of about this weight or heavier tend to be intractable. The author has only had four patients in this category in his present practice.

People in the higher income groups diet with more success as already discussed when considering social aspects (Chap. 4).

A medical reason for losing weight increases the chance of successful weight loss. The successes in such patients in the author's practice more than doubled those who had no medical reason for losing weight (p. 128). It is interesting to note that if the medical reason for losing weight is no longer present, some patients will allow their weight to increase again.

Men are usually more successful than women (Friedman, 1959; Christakis, 1967; Consumers' Association, 1967).

Those who are able and willing to increase appreciably the amount of exercise they take are likely to do well.

The marital state has a beneficial effect upon weight reduction. In the New York series the married subjects were more successful than those who were single and among the author's patients there was a striking difference between childless individuals and those with children, the former rarely being successful dieters (Table XII). Most of those without children were eating to compensate for their lack of a family. It follows that *all those with a strong compulsion to over-eat are likely to do badly.* The extent of this compulsion can be gathered from four simple questions in group 5 of the scheme for assessing the overweight person (p. 112). Those who admit to eating between meals or when depressed or anxious can be given the Shipman A/D Scale (p. 107), which will give a further guide to prognosis.

The patient who has the best chance of dieting successfully, therefore, is a successful business or professional man who has become moderately obese during adult life, is married with children, emotionally mature and with no marked tendency to depression. His success will be quicker if he can take extra exercise and if he has a medical reason for losing weight. Unfortunately less than 10 per cent of the patients with a weight problem who present themselves to a physician come into this category.

Once dieting has started is there any way of assessing the outcome? In the author's practice the response to dieting in the first three months gave a very good indication of the eventual response. Those who are going to do well will lose at the rate of at least $\frac{1}{2}$ kg. (1 lb.) per week during this time. Only five out of 39 patients in Groups I to IV lost less than this, while 13 out of 14 failures (Group V) lost less. Silverstone & Solomon (1965) obtained similar responses to early treatment, and they found that 12 out of 13 successful dieters lost at least 4·5 kg. (10 lb.) in a 13-week period as compared with only four out of 19 failures.

Unfortunately this immediate response is no help in deciding which subjects are likely to relapse and those who will maintain their weight loss, although a guess can usually be made after assessing the factors mentioned earlier.

REFERENCES

CHRISTAKIS, G. (1967). Community programs for weight reduction: experience of the Bureau of Nutrition, New York City. *Can. J. publ. Hlth,* **58,** 499.

CONSUMERS' ASSOCIATION (1967). *Which?,* 5th Oct.

FRIEDMAN, J. (1959). Weight problems and psychological factors. *J. consult. Psychol.* **23,** 524.

GLENNON, J. A. (1966). Weight reduction—an enigma. *Archs intern. Med.* **118,** 1.

SILVERSTONE, J. J. & SOLOMON, T. (1965). The long term management of obesity in general practice. *Br. J. clin. Pract.* **19,** 395.

CHAPTER 13

'Intractable' Obesity

OBESITY resistant to normal methods of treatment by diet and drugs has come to be known as intractable and, in the author's experience, is commonly associated with compensatory eating. The unhappiness and lack of love which often gives rise to the need to eat for compensation is increased by the additional stress of being grossly overweight and the guilt the patient feels when eating in excess, knowing it to be to his detriment.

In each case an attempt should be made to find out the patient's reasons for overeating and his attitude to dieting. If depression is present to any extent, this must be treated (p. 106). If all else fails in patients with intractable obesity, admission to hospital for strict dieting may be the only way of breaking the vicious circle. Nothing short of the loss of 10 to 15 kg. (about 20 to 30 lb.) of excess weight in a few weeks or months is likely to be of much help to the patient with 45 to 70 kg. (about 100 or 150 lb.) of surplus fat. In hospital, fasting is now being used more commonly when other treatments have failed.

Total fasting

The system of total fasting for seven to 10 days in hospital was reported first in 1959 by Bloom in America, confirmed by Duncan (1960) and others in the United States, and in this country by Thomson and his colleagues (1966). The longest follow-up of this type was by Harrison & Marden (1966) from Glasgow who put 62 patients on 10-day fasts and found that 56 of them completed the fast losing an average of 7·4 kg. (16·3 lb.). There was little evidence of hunger and some evidence that their appetites were reduced so that they were more likely to adhere to a low calorie diet than before fasting. A year later 40 per cent of their patients had maintained part of their loss and 4 out of 12 followed up for three years had entirely maintained their weight loss.

Very prolonged fasts recorded include one by Thomson in which 44 kg. (97 lb.) were lost in 236 days. In the U.S.A., Hunscher (1966) from Duncan's clinic reported a follow-up of 709 obese patients who had been fasted in hospital for four to 28 days. Of the 50 per cent who replied, 46 per cent continued to lose weight, and 21 per cent had maintained their weight loss so that two-thirds of those who replied and one-third of the whole series had derived long term benefit from the fast. On the other hand, McCuish, Munro & Duncan (1968) contacted 15 out of 25 patients a year after fasting for 25 days: only one had maintained appreciable weight loss and she became pathologically depressed.

Physiological changes in fasting. There may temporarily be a slight degree of ketosis two or three days after the commencement of fasting. Silverstone et al. (1966) have challenged the view that hunger is absent or reduced in fasting. In nine patients he found that during total starvation for 14 days, hunger was increased during the first day and it then decreased to a normal level. A raised serum uric acid may occur (Drenick et al., 1964) so that fasting is not advised if there is a family or personal history of gout.

Deaths have been reported during fasting for obesity. Cubberley reported in 1965 a case of a 44 year old diabetic patient weighing 180 kg. (396 lb.) who died of lactic acidosis in the ninth week of intermittent fasting when her weight had been reduced by 32 kg. (71 lb.). Spencer (1968) reported two deaths during fasting in patients who commenced to fast while in left ventricular failure.

Only a small part of the weight lost in fasting is fat, most of it being lean body mass. Ball et al. (1967) showed that after 16 days of starvation less than 15 per cent of the weight lost was fat whereas, of the same weight lost by calorie restriction, 70 per cent of the weight lost was fat. This does not apply to prolonged fasting however. Birkenhäger (1968) showed that the fat loss was 60 to 80 per cent of the total weight loss in four patients whose calorie intake averaged 300 cals/day for six to eight weeks. Prolonged fasting must only be undertaken in hospital but, in the author's opinion, fasting for up to ten days is safe in general practice providing an adequate fluid intake is maintained and vitamins are added.

Various other methods of treatment are worthy of trial in patients with intractable obesity as loss of weight, however produced, is of psychological benefit, and several methods should be tried before the expensive alternative of hospital treatment is considered. As they may have metabolic effects both phenformin (p. 82) and fenfluramine (p. 79) should be tried before drug therapy can be said to have failed.

Liquid diets

A balanced liquid diet such as Metercal (Metrecal U.S.A.) taken in equal portions four times daily and providing about 900 calories per day of palatable liquid is useful as a temporary measure to relieve the monotony of dieting. Equally successful for those who like it is Complan powder which has to be mixed with water to make the fluid diet, but is less than half the price. It is almost identical to Metercal in content and, as most housewives dislike spending money on their own diet, it provides a reasonable temporary aid to dieting.

Roberts (1962) from Palm Beach U.S.A. found that 65 out of 78 patients in private practice lost an average of 3·9 kg. (8·6 lb.) in five weeks. Seaton & Duncan (1963) found that 80 per cent of patients lost between 1·8 and 4·1 kg. (4 and 9 lb.) in the first two weeks but the rate of loss dropped rapidly thereafter. In this country 70 out of 82 patients lost an average of 3·2 kg. (7 lb.) in two weeks (General Practitioner Research Group, 1963): 44 were still on the diet after four weeks losing an average of 5·4 kg. (12 lb.), eight remained on the diet for eight weeks losing 9·2 kg. (20·5 lb.) on average. Most patients, therefore, will keep to this diet for two weeks and about 50 per cent of all patients for a month.

Meal substitutes

Bisks, Limmits, Simbix and Trimmetts all contain a low carbohydrate low calorie balanced diet in biscuit form and are intended as substitutes for certain meals or as complete diets. They are only satisfactory for temporary use.

Other modifications of normal dieting

The deadly monotony of permanent dieting can be relieved for many obese patients by going on to special diets for a week or two, or even for as long as one or two months, after which their enthusiasm fades. Most of the special dietary routines advised by magazines are suitable. Seaton & Duncan (1964) tried giving two 500-calorie meals a day to 39 women with refractory obesity; they adhered better to this than to their previous diet and lost an average of 4 kg. (8·9 lb.) in a month. In general, however, most subjects do better with more frequent feeding (p. 38) and Gordon's Diet Plan (p. 54) may well be suitable for long term use by some people as it is more satisfying than most unusual diets.

Frequent injections

A daily injection of chorionic gonadotrophin derived from human pregnancy urine was claimed by Simeons (1954), an Englishman practising in Rome, to produce considerable weight loss in different subjects and Lebon (1961) in this country claimed an average weight loss of about 12·75 kg. (28 lb.) in six weeks for 68 patients by this method. His results provided headlines in one of the national daily papers. Carne (1961), a London general practitioner, showed, however, that similar results could be obtained by using daily injections of saline, *the daily visits to the doctor providing the stimulus for the patient to keep to the 500-calorie diet which was also part of the regime.* In Carne's controlled series patients lost an average of 9·1 kg. (21 lb.) in six weeks with chorionic gonadotrophin and 8·6 kg. (19 lb.) with saline. In a second controlled series they lost 10·1 kg. (22·4 lb.) on the saline injections, and 8 kg. (17·7 lb.) on the diet alone. Those on the diet alone were weighed twice weekly, while those on the injections were weighed and injected six times a week. The daily weighing may perhaps have been more important than the injections. Although there is no statistical proof that these injections are generally effective, it is possible that they are of help in a few cases of obesity. In Lebon's follow-up series of hospital cases (Lebon, 1966) three out of 12 on human chorionic gonadotrophin lost over 9 kg. (20 lb.) in three weeks while two out of 12

on placebo injections lost less than 4·5 kg. (10 lb.), the
remainder of each series losing between 4·5 and 9 kg.

Wine with meals

Lolli (1962), acting on the presumption that most obese
patients have difficulty in controlling their appetite during
the evening, tried allowing 27 of his patients to take a little
wine either before, during or after their evening meal. He
found that the average loss of weight was increased when
patients drank wine *with* their evening meal as compared with
a period of diet excluding alcohol: 14 of his patients lost more
weight on this routine, three lost less and in the remaining
10 the weight loss was the same. It is worth remembering
that Banting's successful diet of over 100 years ago included
wine with meals (p. 46).

Surgery

Plastic surgery. By making a dramatic alteration in a
patient's contour, plastic surgery can raise morale so that
dieting is a much less onerous undertaking. Excessively large
breasts can be reduced with the consequent loss of perhaps
3·2 to 6·4 kg. (7 to 14 lb.) of weight, but the loss of the huge
' apron ' so often found over the abdominal wall in grossly
obese people can produce an immediate loss of up to 25 kg.
(55 lb.) in weight.

By-pass operations. A jejuno-colic shunt to by-pass the
major part of the small intestine and part of the large intestine,
in patients whose lives have been threatened by their bulk,
has been used in the U.S.A. for 10 years. Three deaths have
already been reported as late complications of this operation.
In experimental animals the retained loop is responsible for
their deterioration and this may also apply to humans. This
operation must therefore be regarded as potentially lethal
(*J. Am. med. Ass.*, 1967).

Hypnotherapy

Hypnosis has been tried for most conditions with a strong
psychological element and obesity is no exception. Part of
the success of any measure results from the care with which
a physician takes his patient's history and assesses his social

and psychological background. A good hypnotist uses hypnosis together with other methods of treatment only after a thorough psychological appraisal of the patient's total situation. Hypnotherapy can therefore be expected to help in certain resistant cases of obesity and it has been shown to do so by several authors in America including Hanley (1967) who has recently commenced group hypnotherapy with six to eight women at a time and has found that ' most patients feel that they will be able to maintain their new weight because their attitudes to food have changed, their new eating habits are firmly established and their accomplishments and satisfactions in life preclude the necessity of using food for emotional relief. Patients with a poor prognosis are the very immature who expect hypnosis to accomplish magic with no effort on their part '.

Group therapy

The support of a group of people who understand an individual's problems may give better results than other forms of treatment in a high proportion of obese patients who cannot keep to a diet on their own. James & Christakis (1966) from the New York Health Department, after surveying 2,593 patients from 1953 to 1957 at one of the city's three obesity clinics, found that group treatment which included close supervision by a physician and a nutritionist was more successful than individually supervised weight reduction and they recommend group treatment for all except those suffering from organic and major psychological abnormalities.

An American organisation TOPS (Take Off Pounds Sensibly) has been in existence for over 20 years and has over 185,000 members in U.S.A. and Canada. Most of the 6,000 local chapters of the society are for women only, but there are a small number for men only. There is a strong social element and prizes and awards are given for attaining and maintaining the weight recommended for members by their own physicians. Members are often paired off to help each other and those in difficulty about keeping to their diet can telephone other members for moral support in the same way as can members of Alcoholics Anonymous.

Another American organisation, Weight Watchers, has already enrolled over 6,000 members in over 100 groups in this country. The headquarters are at Weight Watcher House, 2 Thames Street, Windsor, Bucks. Group therapy meetings lasting two hours are held weekly.

A group has been established by the Obesity Association in London (Headquarters, 8 Suffolk Street, London S.W.1.) and others no doubt will follow.

In general practice in this country, Lord (1966) found that group therapy was not successful on a long term basis in his stable rural practice where there were too few new people joining the groups to keep the interest going. Floyd & Ottway (1968; personal communication) in an urban practice have shown that group therapy for periods of six months for each group saves the physician time and gives results comparable with or better than individual therapy. Some patients look forward to their visits and vie with each other as to who shall lose the most weight.

A group of about eight members would appear to be the optimum size and weekly meetings are ideal. In addition to instruction from a nurse or health visitor and/or doctor, some form of social aspect to the group meetings will help to make them more enjoyable. For group therapy in children see p. 172.

Clinics, nursing homes and beauty farms

Many of these places supply group therapy in its most compelling short-term form. Those who can afford private fees are able to lose weight for several weeks under the influence of the discipline, healthy routine and companionship which many of these places provide. The Obesity Association founded in 1967 can advise regarding the quality of establishments in this category. (Secretary, 8 Suffolk Street, London S.W.1.)

ILLUSTRATIVE CASES FROM THE AUTHOR'S
RECENT EXPERIENCE

CASE 1. Mrs. B. was 28 years old, 25 weeks pregnant and weighed 129 kg. (284 lb.). She had been in need of care and protection on account of her mother's loose relationships with men, and was in a residential school for educationally sub-normal pupils for six years, as stress rendered her performance less than her I.Q. of 80. At the age of 21, having had her first illegitimate child she had weighed 100 kg. (222 lb.) and put on weight steadily during her second illegitimate pregnancy and her two subsequent pregnancies, when married to a shiftless irresponsible individual who was in and out of work and prison. At post-natal she weighed 134 kg. (296 lb.) and a year later had stabilised at 133 kg. (294 lb.). She admits openly to eating being one of her few satisfactions in life. More recently she made a great effort and broke the ' 20 stone barrier ', with the help of diethylpropion, to become 120 kg. (236 lb.).

CASE 2. Mrs. E., a widow living with her daughter on whom she was very dependent, was 85·5 kg. (189 lb.) at 69 years of age. She developed ' angina ' whenever the daughter, who was separated from her husband, went out in the evening. The daughter obtained a divorce, remarried and eventually left Mrs. E. living alone in the house. She appeared to be more contented and lost her angina, but her weight increased to 102 kg. (225 lb.) over a period of three years and she admitted to consuming a lot of sugar. With the aid of dexamphetamine followed by phenmetrazine she came down to 99 kg. (208 lb.) in about six months, and later managed to get down to 91 kg. (200 lb.) with further help. At this weight she enjoys her food a great deal but remains active enough to go and baby sit for her married children. She appears to have reached a reasonable compromise with her weight problem.

REFERENCES

BALL, M. F., CANARY, J. J. & KYLE, L. H. (1967). Comparative effects of caloric restriction and metabolic acceleration on body composition in obesity. *Ann. intern. Med.* **67,** 60.

BIRKINHÄGER, J. C. (1968). Changes in body composition during treatment of obesity by intermittent starvation. *Metabolism,* **17,** 391.

BLOOM, W. L. (1959). Fasting as an introduction to the treatment of obesity. *Metabolism,* **8,** 214.

CARNE, S. (1961). The action of chorionic gonadotrophin in the obese. *Lancet,* **2,** 1262.

CORNACCHIA, A. (1967). A layman's view of group therapy in weight control. *Can. J. publ. Hlth,* **58,** 505.

CUBBERLEY, P. T., POLSTER, S. A. & SCHULMAN, C. L. (1965). Lactic acidosis and death after the treatment of obesity by fasting. *New Engl. J. Med.* **272,** 628.

DRENICK, E. J., SWENDSIED, M. E., BLAND, W. H. & TUTTLE, S. C. (1964). Prolonged starvation as treatment for severe obesity. *J. Am. med. Ass.* **187,** 100.

DUNCAN, G., JENSON, W. K., FRASER, R. I. & CHRISTOFORI, F. C. (1960). Correction and control of intractable obesity. Practical applications of intermittent periods of total fasting. *J. Am. med. Ass.* **181,** 309.

GENERAL PRACTITIONER RESEARCH GROUP (1963). Further experience of a dietary product (' metercal ') in selected cases of obesity. *Practitioner,* **190,** 786.

HANLEY, F. W. (1967). The treatment of obesity by individual and group hypnosis. *Can. psychiat. Ass. J.* **12,** 549.

HARRISON, M. T. & MARDEN, R. W. (1966). The long-term value of fasting in the treatment of obesity. *Lancet,* **2,** 1340.

HUNSCHER, M. A. (1966). A post-hospitalisation study of patients treated for obesity by fast regime. *Metabolism,* **15,** 383.

JAMES, G. & CHRISTAKIS, G. (1966). Current programs and research New York City Bureau of Nutrition. *J. Am. Diet. Ass.* **48,** 301.

JOURNAL OF THE AMERICAN MEDICAL ASSOCIATION (1967). Complications of intestinal by-pass for obesity. *Editorial,* **200,** 638.

LEBON, P. (1961). Action of chorionic gonadotrophin in the obese. *Lancet,* **2,** 268.

LEBON, P. (1966). Treatment of overweight patients with chorionic gonadotrophin: follow-up study. *J. Am. Geriat. Soc.* **14,** 116.

LOLLI, C. (1962). The role of wine in the treatment of obesity. *N.Y. St. J. Med.* **62,** 3438.

LORD, W. J. H. (1966). Health education about obesity. *J. Coll. Gen. Practnrs,* **2,** 285.

McCUISH, A. C., MUNRO, J. F. & DUNCAN, L. J. P. (1968). Follow-up study of ' refractory obesity ' treated by fasting. *Br. med. J.* **1,** 91.

ROBERTS, H. J. (1962). Long-term weight reduction in cardiovascular disease. Experiences with a hypocaloric food mixture. *J. Am. Geriat. Soc.* **10,** 308.

SEATON, D. A. & DUNCAN, L. J. P. (1963). Treatment of ' refractory obesity ' with formula diet. *Br. med. J.* **2,** 219.

SEATON, D. A. & DUNCAN, L. J. P. (1964). Treatment of ' refractory obesity ' with a diet of two meals a day. *Lancet,* **2,** 612.

SILVERSTONE, J. T., STARK, J. E. & BUCKLE, R. M. (1966). Hunger during total starvation. *Lancet,* **1,** 1343.

SIMEONS, A. T. W. (1954). The action of chorionic gonadotrophin in the obese. *Lancet,* **2,** 946.

SPENCER, I. O. (1968). Death during therapeutic starvation for obesity. *Lancet,* **1,** 1288.

THOMSON, T. J., RUNCIE, J. & MILLER, V. (1966). Treatment of obesity by total fasting for up to 249 days. *Lancet,* **2,** 992.

CHAPTER 14

Weight Gain in Pregnancy and Its Control

THE six month period during which a pregnant woman attends for ante-natal supervision affords the physician the chance of practising true preventive medicine, the like of which is hard to equal in the whole field of patient/doctor contact in the western world.

Most women when pregnant are health conscious and lessons learnt at this time in their lives will be remembered and passed on to their families. Dietary advice in particular may permanently alter the feeding habits of the whole family.

THE NORMAL WEIGHT GAIN IN PREGNANCY

Chesley (1944) from Jersey City, U.S.A., surveyed in a masterly review 38 papers from the world press starting with Gassner in Munich in 1862 and including all major papers on the subject until 1943. He found that the average weight increase during pregnancy was about 10·9 kg. (24 lb.). In his own personal series of 1,180 patients, the average non-toxaemic gain was 10·6 kg. (23·5 lb.) and he thought that the normal limits of weight gain were that particular figure $\pm$ 4·9 kg. (10·8 lb.), i.e. between 5·8 and 15·5 kg., which is to say, between 12·7 and 34·3 lb. Dieckmann *et al.* (1952) from Chicago give 10·2 kg. (22·6 lb.) as an average non-toxaemic gain and Fish and five other obstetricians in the U.S.A. (1959), surveying 1,000 consecutive cases in private practice, give an average total weight gain of 10·9 kg. (24 lb.). In 1937 Evans wrote the first article on the subject in this country, to be followed by McIlroy & Rodway (1937) who only included from the 24th to the 38th week in their statistics, but used diet control and exercise if weight gain occurred. Scott & Benjamin (1948), published the first detailed British figures in 1948 and in 1,234 cases from local authority clinics they estimated the average weight gain for normotensive patients to be 11·5 kg. (25·25 lb.): 9·6 kg.

(21·25 lb.) from 16 weeks to term and an estimated additional 1·8 kg. (4 lb.) before 16 weeks. Humphreys (1954) gives 11·2 kg. (24·7 lb.) average gain for 1,000 Welsh hospital patients from 12 to 40 weeks, giving an estimated 11·9 kg. (26·2 lb.) for the full term. Thomson & Billewicz (1957) working for the Medical Research Council in Aberdeen give an average of 10 kg. (21·9 lb.) for 1,362 normotensive patients from 13 to 36 weeks, which they estimate as 12·5 kg. (27·6 lb.) for the full pregnancy.

Hytten & Leitch (1964) surveyed 32 papers with information about weight gain in the last two trimesters. Many papers were unacceptable to them as the weight gain had been modified by diet, abnormal pregnancies had been included, or inaccurate estimates had been made of the total weight gain. The only two estimates acceptable to them were those of Humphreys, and Thomson & Billewicz quoted above. They conclude from these two surveys that the normal average weight gain for pregnancy should be 12·5 kg. (27·5 lb.). Is the average the normal however? Lewis (1965) states that about 40 per cent of normal patients show an excess gain in weight of at least twice the average rate at some time in their pregnancy and about 15 per cent gain more than 15·9 kg. (35 lb.). Donald (1966) says that the weight gain should not exceed ' about 28 lb. ', which is about 13 kg., and that Dieckmann's figure of 10·2 kg. (22·6 lb.) is likely to be nearer the normal than is that of Fish or Scott. After discussing the factors contributing to weight gain in pregnancy, and the weight gain during different stages of pregnancy, the author proposes to show that the normal non-toxaemic weight gain should be about 9·5 kg. ± 3·2 kg. (21 lb. ± 7 lb.).

Factors contributing to weight gain in pregnancy

The weight of the uterine contents, the increase in blood volume and the extra cellular fluid can be measured with a fair degree of accuracy, but the increase in weight of the uterus and breasts are estimated and are subject to error.

Weight gain during different stages of pregnancy

The first trimester. Average figures vary greatly in different series, from no weight gain in one series to an average of 1·6 kg.

TABLE XVII

Factors Contributing to Weight Gain in Pregnancy
(From Hytten & Leitch, 1964)

	Average Weight Increase		
	Kg.	(lb.)	
Foetus	3·3	(7·3)	Including blood loss the average
Placenta	0·65	(1·4)	loss at delivery is 5·4 kg. (12 lb.)
Liquor amnii	0·8	(1·8)	(McIlroy).
Uterus	0·9	(2·0)	
Breasts	0·4	(0·9)	
Blood (increase in volume)	1·25	(2·7)	Average loss early puerperium
Extracellular fluid	1·2	(2·6)	2·4 kg. (5·2 lb.) (McIlroy).

The weight unaccounted for is mainly fat.   *Total weight gain*

The author's estimate allows for 1·3 kg. (2·8 lb.)   9·8 kg. (21·5 lb.)
Hytten & Leitch allow for . . 4 kg. (8·8 lb.)   12·5 kg. (27·5 lb.)

(3·5 lb.) in another. Factors causing variation are the stage of pregnancy at first attendance, the incidence of vomiting and the presence or absence of dietary advice at this stage. Few English series have many recordings of weights at eight or nine weeks in addition to 12 or 13 weeks but there appears to be no justification for taking Cumming's figure (1934) of 0·25 kg. (0·5 lb.) total gain as normal, as has been done by both Humphreys (1954) and Dawson & Borg (1949). Hytten & Leitch (1964) take Chelsey's figure (1944) of 1·1 kg. (2·5 lb.) as ' consistent with clinical experience and not likely to be far out '. All the author's patients who have had two recordings during the first trimester have gained from 0·255 (0·5 lb.) to 2·7 kg. (6 lb.) in weight, and he has taken 0·9 kg. (2 lb.) as the normal weight gain and considered 1·8 kg. (4 lb.) or over as an indication for dietary control.

The second trimester. The American figures vary between 3·6 and 6·6 kg. (8·0 and 14·6 lb.) but Dieckmann *et al.,* whose figures are more reliable and authoritative than most, give an average of about 4 kg. (9 lb.). Average figures from Local Authority clinics (Scott & Benjamin, 1948) show 4 kg. (8·9 lb.) for the weeks 16 to 24, as against 3·3 kg. (7·4 lb.) for the next eight weeks. This would average about 6·2 kg. (13·6 lb.) for the 13 weeks: Humphrey's average for 1,000 hospital patients was 6·2 kg. (13·7 lb.). Most of the author's patients needing dietary advice were given it during this trimester. The author regards a total gain of 2·2 kg. (4·9 lb.) for the weeks 13 to 20 as normal and 3·4 kg. (7·5 lb.) for the weeks 20 to 30, which averages 4·3 kg. (9·5 lb.) for the weeks 13 to 26. A gain of 1·8 kg. (4 lb.) in four weeks up to 20 weeks has been regarded as abnormal and a more rapid gain than that as excessive in any subsequent four week period.

TABLE XVIII

Estimated Average Normal Weight Gain in Pregnancy

Weeks	Gain per week		Total weight gain	
	kg.	(lb.)	kg.	(lb.)
9 - 13	0·23	(0·5)	0·9	(2·0)
13 - 20	0·32	(0·7)	2·3	(4·9)
20 - 30	0·34	(0·75)	3·4	(7·5)
30 - 40	0·32	(0·7)	3·2	(7·0)
Total			9·8	(21·4)

The third trimester. Here there is more general agreement as to the average weight gain in non-toxaemic cases and many series give figures between 4 and 5 kg. (9 and 11 lb.). In this country McIlroy & Rodway (1937) give 4·4 kg. (9·7 lb.) and Scott & Benjamin 4·3 kg. (9·4 lb.). The author regards 4·5 kg. (10·0 lb.) as average in non-toxaemic cases (14 weeks).

10

The author's series

This is a retrospective survey of the last 100 pregnant women who attended the ante-natal clinic held weekly in the author's consulting rooms, who were weighed regularly from before the 20th week of pregnancy (81 before the 16th week) until the 36th week or later, and who still remained in the practice; 50 were primiparae and 50 multiparae. A further 69 women were seen ante-natally during the course of the survey, but were delivered in hospital and were not seen as late as the 36th week by him, or were not weighed over a long enough period.

Scott & Benjamin showed quite clearly that the initial weight has little bearing on the rate of weight increase and in fact their heaviest group who started a pregnancy weighing over 76 kg. (12 stone) gained less weight on average than those whose commencing weight was under that figure. Humphreys (1954) confirmed these findings. When discussing the weight gain throughout pregnancy therefore, the initial weight has been discounted when making comparisons between groups of patients. An average normal weight gain has been added for missed weeks where necessary to estimate the total gain from eight or nine weeks to 40 weeks (Table XVIII).

As 60 of the 100 women gained excessive weight before the last trimester of their pregnancy, and six of the remaining 40 were toxaemic, only 34 can be regarded as ' normal '. All 34 fell within the range of 6·4 to 12·75 kg. (14 to 28 lb.) having an average gain of 9·75 (21·4 lb.) with the exception of five women in all of whom there were special circumstances.

One of these was overweight at the beginning of pregnancy and gained only 4·5 kg. (10 lb.). Another gained only 4·75 kg. (10·5 lb.) but vomited during most of her pregnancy. Two others, following a recent attack of influenza, were underweight at the beginning of pregnancy and regained their normal weight during pregnancy thereby gaining gross weights of 14 kg. (31 lb.) and 15·4 kg. (34 lb.) respectively. The fifth woman gained 14 kg. (31 lb.) in her first pregnancy and only 9·75 kg. (21·5 lb.) in her second. As the weight at the beginning of each pregnancy was the same and she did not need to diet in either, fluid retention probably accounted for the excessive weight gain in the first pregnancy.

The author also assessed 23 further pregnancies undergone within this group of 100 women, for the incidence of toxaemia.

DIETARY ADVICE DURING PREGNANCY

Almost unbelievable results have been obtained by strict dietary control in the past. Hannah (1925) in America aimed at a weight gain of only 6·4 kg. (14 lb.) and in 236 private cases whom he weighed weekly throughout pregnancy, he was able to achieve his aim by a low carbohydrate low fat diet, the total average weight gain being only 6 kg. (13·25 lb.) while 25 patients (1·5 per cent) actually lost weight; in spite of this the average weight of the babies was 3·2 kg. (7·13 lb.). Slemons & Fagan (1927) dieted their patients strictly, allowing no milk at all after quickening, to produce an average weight gain of 7·5 kg. (16·5 lb.) in 500 cases. Hamlin (1952), in Australia, aimed at limiting weight gain to 3·6 kg. (8 lb.) between the 20th and 30th week of pregnancy but the author could find no series in the literature giving the results of selective dieting for those gaining weight in early pregnancy.

The author's series

In the present series 60 cases required dietary advice for obesity. Eight of these were dieted at the onset of pregnancy, a total of 56 before the 24th week and four from the 24th to the 30th weeks. Nine of these women were thin at the start of pregnancy. Those who were not obese at the start of pregnancy and in a four weekly period gained 1·8 kg. (4 lb.) or more before 20 weeks, or over 1·8 kg. between 20 and 30 weeks were advised as to their diet. Each woman was told that there were two reasons for avoiding excessive weight gain in pregnancy. The first reason was that she was likely to think that her increasing weight was merely due to the pregnancy, but that in fact it was due to fat, and she would be very disappointed when she found that she could not find any clothes to fit her after her lying-in period. In most cases the author was able to demonstrate the presence of excess adipose tissue without difficulty by clinical assessment of skinfold thickness. The second reason was that excessive weight gain during pregnancy could be harmful to her baby.

Results of treatment. In assessing the results of treatment, the author regarded as a successful response to diet a lesser gain in weight than normal during the subsequent four weeks, and as a partially successful response a reduced rate of weight gain. In 46 cases an enquiry was made about the individual's dietary habits and detailed advice was given concerning a

TABLE XIX

Results of Dietary Treatment in 60 Cases of Weight Gain in Pregnancy

	No. of Patients 1.	Av. wt. in lbs. before diet 2.	Correc- ted gain 3.	Av. gain after dieting 4.	Correc- ted loss 5.	Wt. swing 6.
Given Dietary Advice	46					
Successful	33	5·7	3·2	0·3	2·7	−5·9
Gained less weight	7	5·4	2·7	3·7	+1·5	−1·2
Gained less or failed (trans- ferred to diet)	5	4·3	1·9	3·8	+1·0	−0·9
Failed	1	2·8	1·5	5·5	+2·3	+0·8
Diet Sheet given	19					
Successful after transfer	5	3·8	1·0	−1·3	4·3	−5·3
Dieted initially	14					
Successful	13	6·1	3·5	−0·2	2·7	−6·2
Failed	1	5·5	2·7	6·0	+2·9	+0·2
Summary of Successes	51	5·7	3·1	−0·1	2·9	−6·0

The weight gains in columns 2 to 5 inclusive are standardised to periods of 4 weeks each.

reduction of carbohydrate intake. Success occurred in 33 cases, in 10 cases the rate of weight gain lessened, and three cases were failures. To two of these failures, to three who gained less weight than previously and to an additional 14 patients a written diet was given (modified Marriott, p. 52, with the daily milk ration increased to one pint). All except one responded successfully (Table XIX).

Summary

Lost weight (corrected)	51	(18 achieved gross weight loss)
Gained less weight	7	
Failed to lose weight	2	

The one complete failure was a woman who had a duodenal ulcer and also ran a small home for elderly women for whom she had to do all the cooking. She gained a total of 16·75 kg. (37 lb.) during the pregnancy. One other patient, who was slim at the beginning of pregnancy, gained a total of 13·1 kg. (29 lb.) from the 6th to the 40th week; she failed to respond to dietary advice, but was not put on to a stricter diet.

The 51 women who lost weight did extremely well in that the corrected weight gain of an average of 1·4 kg. (3·1 lb.) in one four weekly period was converted to a corrected weight loss of 1·3 kg. (2·9 lb.) in the subsequent four weeks, a difference in one month of 2·7 kg. (6 lb.) as compared with the previous month. Only one of these patients was given an anorectic drug: she had always found great difficulty in weight control and was under considerable stress at the time.

The eight women who were obese at the beginning of pregnancy and were put on a diet immediately, included one case of toxaemia. The remaining seven gained an average of only 8·5 kg. (18·7 lb.), thereby losing a little of their initial fat. This is almost identical with Mullins' results (p. 158).

As a result of the dietary advice given the overall average weight gain of the 60 who were dieted was 10·6 kg. (23·4 lb.) compared with the average weight gain of 9·75 kg. (21·4 lb.) of those who were not dieted. *Excluding toxaemic cases the corrected weight gain for the 49 dieters was only 10 kg. (22·2 lb.), or less than 0·45 kg. (1 lb.) more than the average of 9·75 kg. (21·4 lb.) for the 34 non-toxaemic cases who did not*

require to diet. Only two patients in the whole series, one of whom was toxaemic, gained more than 15·8 kg. (35 lb.) as against Lewis's estimate (1965) of 15 per cent of normal patients (p. 143) and Fish's figure (1959) of 9·8 per cent. Seven of the 14 who gained more than 12·75 kg. (28 lb.) were toxaemic.

TABLE XX

Weight Gains in 100 Pregnancies

	No.	Average weight gain	
		kg.	(lb.)
Non-toxaemic women not dieted (normal)	34	9·7	(21·4)
Toxaemic women not dieted	6	9·9	(21·7)
Non-toxaemic women dieted	49	10·1	(22·2)
Toxaemic women dieted	11	13·6	(30·0)
Total non-toxaemic	83	10·0	(21·9)
Total toxaemic	17	12·3	(27·1)
Complete series	100	10·3	(22·6)
Gained over 28 lb.	14 (7 toxaemic)		
Gained over 35 lb.	2 (1 toxaemic)		

DISCUSSION

Hytten and Leitch consider that the average weight gain of 12·5 kg. (27·5 lb.) in two series should be regarded as the normal weight gain and they estimate that this includes 4 kg. (8·8 lb.) of fat. They justify this large amount of ' fat store ' which is mainly accumulated in the first thirty weeks, by presuming that in women who work throughout pregnancy it is needed as a buffer against possible food deprivation in the later weeks of pregnancy. Members of their own group, however (Thomson *et al.*, 1966), found that the average weight gain of rural African women varied with the season of the year from 2·2 to 5·3 kg. (4·9 to 11·7 lb.). Of the 60 of the author's who were advised to lose weight, the 51 who succeeded in losing most of the fat they had accumulated did so on a free diet in which there was merely restriction of carbohydrate, and in some cases moderate restriction of fat in addition. No calorie control whatever was practised.

The increased oestrogen output of pregnancy resulting in an impairment of carbohydrate tolerance leads to an increased fat synthesis, therefore only in the presence of an excessive carbohydrate intake.

It appears illogical, therefore, that the average accumulation of fat is in fact excessive and that the author's figure of 9·7 kg. (21·4 lb.) is more likely to be normal than the figure of 12·5 kg. (27·5 lb.) which includes 4 kg. (8·8 lb.) of fat.

WEIGHT GAIN IN RELATION TO TOXAEMIA

There has been much misunderstanding about this subject because of confusion between the two main causes of weight gain, i.e. simple obesity and fluid retention. In the author's experience evidence of excessive gain in weight due to excessive calorie intake is usually shown before the 26th week of pregnancy, while in most cases of fluid retention weight gain is not shown until after this and in many it is sudden in onset.

According to Chesley (1944), Zangemeister in 1916 was the first obstetrician to correlate weight gain in pregnancy with toxaemia. Hannah (1925) used his very strict weight control and weekly surveillance mainly in an attempt to reduce the incidence of eclampsia which had occurred in three of his 236 cases in a previous pregnancy. Siddall & Mack (1938) put the correlation on a more scientific basis. In 100 cases of toxaemia, they found that 61 had doubled the average weight gain at some time in the last trimester and in 37 of these the weight gain preceded a rise in blood pressure. Thus in over one-third of all their toxaemic cases an earlier sign than a rise in blood pressure had been found.

In this country Evans (1937) found that out of 211 patients, 41 gained more than 3·6 kg. (8 lb.) in a month; 26 of these (63 per cent) became toxaemic later; of 101 without any abnormal weight gain only one became toxaemic. McIlroy &

Rodway found that between 24 to 28 weeks, toxic cases gained an average of 2·1 kg. (4·7 lb.) and non-toxic 1·61 kg. (3·55 lb.).

Like so many important advances in medicine it was many years before the profession as a whole took enough notice to modify its routine treatment accordingly. It was not until Hamlin of Sydney published his classical retrospective survey in the *Lancet* in 1952 that the control of weight gain in middle and late pregnancy for prevention of toxaemia began to affect the general practice of obstetrics.

Hamlin found that if the weight gain from the 20th to the 30th weeks was 3·6 kg. (8 lb.) or less in young primigravidae no pre-eclamptic toxaemia ensued. Oedema of the fingers at 31 weeks was almost invariably followed by a raised blood pressure at 37 or 38 weeks. Incipient oedema was treated by a high protein, low carbohydrate, salt restricted diet, and patients were seen weekly or every fourth day. In 1945-7 there had been 28 cases of eclampsia (1/500 bookings) which Hamlin compared with a rate of 1/600 at the Rotunda (Dublin) in 1836. With his new routine there were no cases whatever in 1948 to 1952.

It may be that different factors operate in Australia from the British Isles, as in Thomson's Aberdeen series (1957), 73 per cent of normotensives gained more than 3·6 kg. (8 lb.) from 20 to 30 weeks (85 per cent of P.E.T.). Nevertheless he found an increasing difference in weight gain between non-toxic cases, those with a rise in blood pressure and those with albuminuria in addition.

TABLE XXI

Average Weight Gains in the Toxaemias Compared with the Normal (Thomson 1967)

Type of Case	Number	Average Weight Gains per Week		
		13 - 20/52	20 - 30/52	30 - 36/52
		kg. (lb.)	kg. (lb.)	kg. (lb.)
P.E.T. with albuminuria	166	0·45 (1·0)	0·56 (1·23)	0·68 (1·50)
Hypertensive	533	0·43 (0·95)	0·52 (1·14)	0·49 (1·08)
Normal	1362	0·42 (0·92)	0·46 (1·03)	0·39 (0·87)

These Aberdeen findings paralleled those of Dieckmann *et al.* in the U.S.A. Thomson found that the incidence of eclampsia in Aberdeen dropped from 8/1,000 (1938-42) to 2/1,000 in 1954-5 and later to 0·8/1,000 without any weight control. The main factor responsible for the improvement in these figures was probably better ante-natal care. This also is the likely reason why Hamlin produced such a dramatic improvement in the Sydney figures, rather than his insistence on weight control. Theobald (1962) in Bradford examined his patients weekly from the 24th week onwards and increased his ante-natal intake by cutting post-natal stay in hospital. By these means he reduced the number of cases of eclampsia from 71 in 1947-51 to seven in 1956-61 (0·02 per cent in 35,000 deliveries) and no mother or baby was lost from this cause.

McGillivray (1961) found that in 4,215 primigravidae, toxaemia usually occurred if the weight gain between the 20th and 30th week was over 0·56 kg. (1·25 lb.) per week. He stated that eclampsia could only be prevented by noting a sudden gain in weight. Rhodes (1962) confirmed the increased weight gain in mild toxaemic cases (46) as compared with normal (50 cases) but found a decreased weight gain in eclampsia (29 cases from three hospitals).

The author's series

Defining toxaemia as a rise in blood pressure to a diastolic level of 90 on two occasions occurring after the 26th week of pregnancy (McGillivray, 1961) there were 13 cases of toxaemia in the 100 pregnancies and 15 in the larger series of 123 pregnancies. In four other cases in the main series and one in the larger series toxaemia probably occurred although the diastolic blood pressure never rose to 90. In each case there was a sudden weight increase which responded rapidly to rest and salt restriction, and in addition in four of the five cases the diastolic blood pressure was raised to 10 or 15 mm. above the patient's normal. This brings the total of toxaemic cases to 17 (10 primiparae) in the main series and 20 altogether. *In 14 of these 20 cases there was a sudden rise in weight detected between the 27th and 38th weeks.* In seven cases a rise in diastolic blood pressure was shown at the same time (Fig. 11) but *in seven cases the sudden weight gain preceded the rise in blood*

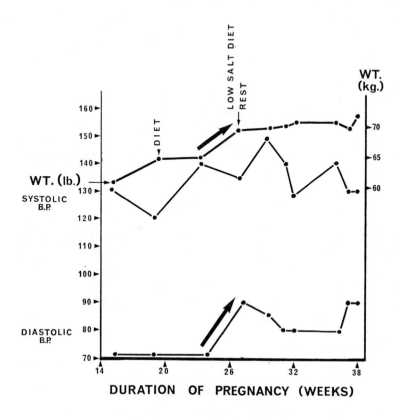

FIG. 11

SUDDEN WEIGHT GAIN AT THE SAME TIME AS RISE IN B.P.

pressure by from one to eight weeks (Fig. 12). The sudden onset of the rise is emphasized in Table XXII as is the dramatic response to treatment.

Of the remaining six cases four showed evidence of excessive increase in adipose tissue before the 24th week and responded initially to diet, following which they recommenced a steady weight gain, probably due to fluid retention (Fig. 13).

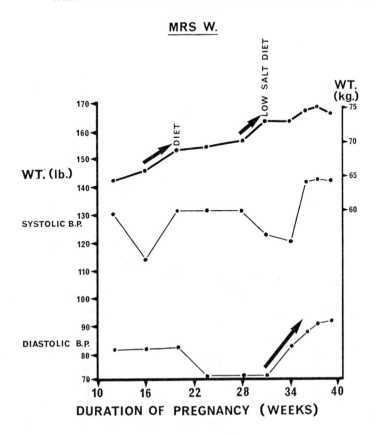

SUDDEN WEIGHT GAIN
PRECEDING RISE IN B.P.

Fig. 12

Figures 11, 12 and 13 illustrate the importance of the diastolic blood pressure and the relative unimportance of the
systolic pressure.

It will be seen from Table XXI that the toxaemic cases
gained on average 2·4 kg. (5·2 lb.) which is 23·7 per cent more
than the non-toxaemic cases although more than half of them
(10/17) gained 12·75 kg. (28 lb.) or under.

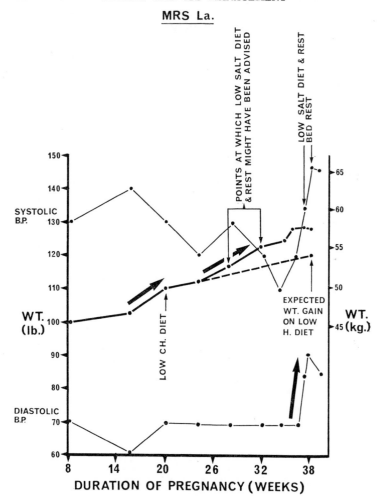

STEADY EXCESSIVE WEIGHT
GAIN DUE TO FLUID RETENTION

Fig. 13

Differentiation between the causes of weight gain

In most cases, the differentiation between the increase in weight due to simple obesity and that due to fluid retention associated with toxaemia, is not difficult if careful attention is paid to the pattern of weight gain. As previously stated, all

TABLE XXII
Rate of Gain Before, During and After Sudden Rise in Weight

Average Weekly Weight Gain between two consecutive readings	Weight Gain per Week			
	Dieted (8)		Not Dieted (6)	
	kg.	(lb.)	kg.	(lb.)
Before sudden rise in weight	0·14	(0·3)	0·36	(0·8)
During sudden rise in weight	0·72	(1·6)	0·81	(1·8)
After sudden rise in weight	−0·36	(−0·8)	−0·26	(−0·5)

60 patients in the main series who needed advice regarding obesity showed evidence of excessive weight gain by the 26th week and 57 of them by the 24th week.

Of these women 11 developed toxaemia later and showed a further gain in weight due to fluid retention at 27 weeks or later. Eight suddenly increased in weight and three did so gradually after having previously lost weight on a diet. Two others in the series followed similar patterns to these three but did not proceed to toxaemia, and the secondary rise in weight during the third trimester was due to a relapse of dietary control and not to fluid retention. In each case the diastolic blood pressure when the secondary rise occurred was lower than at the previous reading.

In four toxaemic cases where weight gain had been within normal limits previously, a sudden gain in weight occurred after the 27th week. Thus out of a total of 64 women who gained excessively during pregnancy five gained gradually after having previously lost weight on a low carbohydrate diet. In three of these the passage of time was necessary to elucidate the cause of the weight increase, but in the remaining 61 patients there was no real difficulty if the weight and blood pressure changes were carefully assessed at each attendance.

It is likely that in those cases where there was some difficulty in deciding the cause of weight increase there was some fluid retention before 26 weeks in addition to fat, as Hytten *et al.* (1966) have shown that in women who develop generalised oedema either with or without toxaemia late in pregnancy, fluid retention begins at about the 20th week. In all other women fluid retention begins at about the 30th week.

SUMMARY: In the second trimester weight gain is almost invariably due to simple obesity. In the third trimester, sudden weight gain is due to the fluid retention of toxaemia, but if weight gain is gradual, after previously successful dieting, differentiation may be difficult unless the blood pressure readings provide a lead.

THE EFFECTS OF EXCESSIVE WEIGHT GAIN IN PREGNANCY

Effect on the mother. The end result of a lack in dietary control can be devastating in its effect on the individual mother and her family. The classic case quoted by Richardson (1952) was a 44·5 kg. (7 stone) primigravida who was 5 kg. (11 lb.) underweight at the beginning of her first pregnancy. Her weight increased with each of her six pregnancies and she ended up weighing 111 kg. (17 st. 7 lb.), a total increase in weight of 150 per cent.

Nine out of Richardson's 39 patients who became obese during pregnancy were in fact underweight initially, as were nine of the author's 60 like subjects who needed dietary advice. Moreover, two of these nine had difficulty in maintaining their weight when not pregnant, which shows that *being underweight normally is no guarantee that obesity will not develop during pregnancy.*

Effects on the foetus. The effects of unbridled weight gain can also be disastrous to the foetus. Richardson's and Sheldon's (1949) figures combined show a total perinatal mortality in 80 obese women of 11/208 (5·3 per cent) and only 3/200 (1·5 per cent) in 70 controls. Mullins (1960) looked after 35 obese multiparae referred to her from the ante-natal clinics. The 25 looked after throughout pregnancy gained an average of 8 kg. (18 lb.) compared with 27 kg. (59 lb.) in previous pregnancies when their weight had been uncontrolled, and 22 kg. (49 lb.) when weight gain had been supervised in the ante-natal clinic. All ended in the normal delivery of a healthy infant, but in the previous 43 pregnancies there had been five stillbirths, six forceps deliveries, three caesarian sections and eight cases of toxaemia. More recently Thomson & Billewicz (1957) found that from the 20th to 36th week of pregnancy 5·4 to 7·25 kg. (12 to 16 lb.) weight gain (0·34 to 0·45 kg., or 0·75 to 1 lb., per week average) gave the lowest figures for perinatal mortality (11·9 per 1,000 out of 1,090 cases). A gain of 7·25 to 9·1 kg. (16 to 20 lb.) at the rate of 0·45 to 0·56 kg. (1 to 1·25 lb.) per week led to the figures being more than doubled (27·8 per 1,000 out of 1,009 cases) and a gain of over 9·1 kg. (20 lb.), which is more than 0·56 kg. (1·25 lb.) per week, led to trebling of the incidence (32·9 per 1,000 out of 1,124 cases).

There was no perinatal mortality in the author's series of 123 pregnancies.

THE EFFECTS OF OBESITY AT THE ONSET OF PREGNANCY

Excessive weight gain in one pregnancy commonly leads to obesity at the beginning of the next, and obesity at the onset of pregnancy gives rise to an increased risk of developing toxaemia. Tompkins *et al.* (1955) in the U.S.A. found 4·2 per cent cases of toxaemia in 237 women who were 20 per cent overweight compared with 2·2 per cent in 1,263 women within the range of plus or minus 20 per cent of normal weight. In this country Williams (1957) found the initial weight in 50 cases of toxaemia averaged 61·8 kg. (136·4 lb.) compared with that of 50 normal cases weighing only 58·5 kg. (129·1 lb.). Emerson (1962) found 4 per cent of 626 patients of normal weight developed toxaemia and 19 per cent of 231 patients who were overweight. The foetal loss in the normals was 2·1 per cent and in the overweight 8·7 per cent.

THE LONG TERM RESULTS OF DIETARY ADVICE IN PREGNANCY

Weight control. For dietary advice during pregnancy to prove truly effective it should result in a woman's weight being the same or less than originally, at the start of her next pregnancy. 29 patients in the series were weighed at the start of their next pregnancies; 15 had lost at least 1·3 kg. (3 lb.) while seven had gained weight. Those who had dieted fared better than those who had not, 12 out of 21 having lost weight compared with three out of eight.

The weight at the commencement of a subsequent pregnancy is a better guide than the weight at post-natal examination, as some patients continued to lose weight afterwards. Out of 12 of the author's patients who were weighed at post-natal and again at the start of the next pregnancy 10 had lost an average of 1·8 to 2·25 kg. (4 to 5 lb.). In some cases the knowledge that her post-natal weight was found to be above her pre-natal weight may have assisted a woman in bringing about this loss.

Toxaemia. The incidence of toxaemia in pregnancy is increased by weight gain and also by being overweight at the onset of pregnancy.

The control of weight gain due to obesity in the second trimester is likely, therefore, to lead to a reduction in the overall incidence of toxaemia and thereby to a reduction in perinatal morbidity.

SUMMARY OF THE AUTHOR'S RESEARCH

1. 100 consecutive ante-natal patients with complete weight records prior to the 20th week of pregnancy until after the 36th week have been assessed in detail. In addition, 23 have been followed through a subsequent pregnancy.
2. Evidence is given to show that the *normal* weight gain in pregnancy should be 9·5 kg. (21 lb.) plus or minus 3·2 kg. (7 lb.) and not the *average* weight gain of 12·5 kg. (27·5 lb.) in previous British series.
3. To 60 patients dietary advice was given regarding their excessive weight increase noted by the end of the second trimester. On a low carbohydrate, free calorie diet 51 lost weight (corrected) and 7 gained less weight than previously. As a result of dieting, the average total weight gain during pregnancy, excluding toxaemic cases, was less than 0·45 kg. (1 lb.) more than in normal cases, and only two gained more than 15·8 kg. (35 lb.). A strong case has been made for the giving of dietary advice to any woman who gains 1·8 kg. (4 lb.) per month before the 20th week or 2·25 kg. (5 lb.) per month in any successive four weekly period thereafter.
4. Weight gain occurring during the third trimester is usually due to the fluid retention associated with toxaemia. The 17 cases of mild to moderate toxaemia occurring in 100 pregnancies gained an average of 2·4 kg. (5·2 lb.) more than the non-toxaemic cases. *Of the 20 cases of toxaemia in the larger series of 123 pregnancies 14 showed a characteristic sudden weight gain which responded dramatically to rest*

and salt restriction. In seven cases the sudden gain in weight was the earliest sign of toxaemia, preceding a rise in blood pressure by from one to eight weeks. Weight gain in itself is a useful sign even though it occurs frequently without other signs of toxaemia, provided that a differentiation is made between weight gain due to the laying down of fat which occurs usually in the second trimester and weight gain due to retention of fluid which occurs usually in the third trimester.

REFERENCES

CHESLEY, L. C. (1944). Weight changes and water balance in normal and toxic pregnancy. *Am. J. Obstet. Gynec.* **48,** 565.

CHESLEY, L. C. & CHESLEY, E. M. (1943). An analysis of some factors associated with the development of pre-eclampsia. *Am. J. Obstet. Gynec.* **45,** 748.

CUMMINGS, H. H. (1934). An interpretation of weight changes during pregnancy. *Am. J. Obstet. Gynec.* **27,** 808.

DAWSON, Sir B. & BORG, H. (1949). Increase of weight during pregnancy. *N.Z. med. J.* **48,** 357.

DIECKMANN, W. J., SMITTER, R. C. & RYNKIEWICZ, L. (1952). Pre-eclampsia-eclampsia does not cause permanent vascular-renal disease. *Am. J. Obstet. Gynec.* **64,** 850.

DONALD, I. (1966). *Practical Obstetric Problems.* 3rd Ed. London: Lloyd-Luke.

EMERSON, R. G. (1962). Obesity and its association with the complications of pregnancy. *Br. med. J.* **2,** 516.

EVANS, M. D. A. (1937). Variations of weight during pregnancy. *Br. med. J.* **1,** 157.

FISH, J. S., BARTHOLOMEW, R. A., COLVIN, E. G., GRIMES, W. H., LESTER, W. M. & GALLOWAY, W. H. (1959). The relationship of pregnancy weight gain to toxaemia. *Am. J. Obstet. Gynec.* **78,** 743.

HANNAH, C. R. (1925). Weight during pregnancy with observations and statistics. *Am. J. Obstet. Gynec.* **9,** 854.

HAMLIN, R. H. J. (1952). The prevention of eclampsia and pre-eclampsia. *Lancet,* **1,** 64.

HUMPHREYS, R. C. (1954). An analysis of the maternal and foetal weight factor in normal pregnancy. *J. Obstet. Gynaec. Br. Emp.* **61,** 765.

HYTTEN, F. E. & LEITCH, J. (1964). *The Physiology of Human Pregnancy.* Oxford: Blackwell.

HYTTEN, F. E., THOMSON, A. M. & TAGGART, N. (1966). Total body water in normal pregnancy. *J. Obstet. Gynaec. Br. Commonw.* **73,** 553.

KERR, M. G. (1962). The problem of the overweight patient in pregnancy. *J. Obstet. Gynaec. Brit. Emp.* **69,** 988.

LEWIS, T. L. T. (1965). *Progress in Clinical Obstetrics and Gynaecology.* 2nd Ed. London: Churchill.

MACGILLIVRAY, I. (1961). Hypertension in pregnancy and its consequences. *J. Obstet. Gynaec. Br. Emp.* **68,** 557.

MCILROY, A. L. & RODWAY, H. E. (1937). Weight changes during and after pregnancy. *J. Obstet. Gynaec. Br. Emp.* **44,** 221.

MULLINS, A. (1960). Overweight in Pregnancy. *Lancet,* **1,** 146.

RHODES, P. (1962). The significance of weight gain in pregnancy. *Lancet,* **1,** 663.

RICHARDSON, J. S. (1952). The treatment of maternal obesity. *Lancet,* **1,** 525.

SCOTT, J. H. & BENJAMIN, B. (1948). Weight changes in pregnancy. *Lancet,* **1,** 550.

11

SHELDON, J. H. (1949). Maternal obesity. *Lancet,* **2,** 869.

SIDDALL, R. S. & MACK, H. E. (1938). Weight changes and toxaemia of late pregnancy. *Am. J. Obstet. Gynec.* **36,** 380.

SLEMONS, J. H. & FAGAN, R. H. (1927). A study of the infant birth weight and the mother's gain during pregnancy. *Am. J. Obstet. Gynec.* **14,** 159.

STEWART, A. M. (1959). Environmental hazards of pregnancy. *J. Obstet. Gynaec. Br. Emp.* **66,** 739.

THEOBALD, G. W. (1962). Weekly antenatal care and home on the second day. *Lancet,* **1,** 735.

THOMSON, A. M., BILLEWICZ, W. Z., THOMSON, P. & MACGREGOR, I. A. (1966). Body weight changes during pregnancy and lactation in rural African (Gambian) women. *J. Obstet. Gynaec. Br. Commonw.* **73,** 724.

THOMSON, A. M. & BILLEWICZ, W. Z. (1957). Clinical significance of weight trends during pregnancy. *Br. med. J.* **1,** 243.

THOMSON, A. M., HYTTEN, F. E. & BILLEWICZ, W. Z. (1967). The epidemiology of oedema during pregnancy. *J. Obstet. Gynec. Br. Commonw.* **74,** 1.

TOMPKINS, W. J., WIEHL, D. G. & MITCHELL, R. McN. (1955). The underweight patients as an increased obstetric hazard. *Am. J. Obstet. Gynec.* **69,** 114.

WILLIAMS. C. D. (1957). Weight in relation to pregnancy toxaemia. *Br. med. J.* **2,** 1338.

CHAPTER 15

Obesity in Childhood

THE clinical estimation of obesity in children is no more difficult than in adults, but the assessment of weight change is not too easy owing to the changes occurring during normal growth. The incidence of obesity in childhood is hard to assess but it is likely to be between 5 and 15 per cent in this country. It was 8 per cent in adolescent girls in Croydon (Mortimer, 1968).

THE NORMAL GROWTH PATTERN

This has been clarified recently by Tanner and his associates (1966) who have shown that the rate of normal growth is approximately doubled during puberty for about a year, the peak weight velocity following closely on the peak height velocity. In boys the peak height velocity occurring at the age of 14 is about 10 cm. per year (range 7 to 15 cm.) and the peak weight velocity is nearly 10 kg. (22 lb.) per year with a range of 5 to 14 kg. (11 to 30 lb.). In girls the peak height velocity occurs at about 12 years of age averaging about 9 cm. a year (range 6 to 11 cm.) and the peak weight velocity follows at nearly 13 years of age when it is almost 9 kg., or about 20 lb. per year with a range of 5 to 14 kg (11 to 30 lb.).

Grant (1966) from a nine-year survey of 740 children found that obesity developed if the weight gain was more than 10 per cent per two inches gained in height. If this rate persisted for eight years the child would not ' grow out of ' the state of obesity.

AETIOLOGY

Hormonal causes are rare and can be ruled out for practical purposes.

Hereditary tendencies. Strong hereditary tendencies exist in many obese children and the stronger they are, the earlier in life will they show, and therefore in most children with an early tendency to obesity the hereditary element is well marked.

163

As previously stated it exhibits itself in most individuals as a general slowness of movement and a liking for food. Obese children as a rule have less food dislikes than other children and have a preference for carbohydrate foods, especially those containing sugar.

Emotional factors. In addition to hereditary tendencies there is a large emotional element in many cases. Food is of paramount importance in a child's life: apart from sleeping, the intake of food is a baby's main occupation and is associated with contact with the mother. As the child's personality develops from the age of 18 months to three years, food often provides a source of friction. A child soon learns that to refuse food may give him a sense of power over his parents. Food of which he is especially fond is commonly given for reward and withheld for punishment. Unhappy children often eat from lack of affection, and mothers often press food on them because they realise subconsciously that they don't love them enough. As a result of lack of affection in infancy and early childhood, many obese children mature slowly and are therefore tied emotionally to their mothers for longer than average.

An important study by Bruch & Touraine (1940) of 40 obese children and their family backgrounds represented a 25 per cent cross section of the 160 children under their surveillance at Columbia University. They described the children as ' overprotected, unhelpful, inactive and disinterested '. The fathers were mainly weak and unaggressive persons and the mothers had suffered from poverty and insecurity. Only in a few families was the marital relationship satisfactory; 70 per cent of the children were the only children or the youngest and more than 50 per cent had been unwanted. Excessive feeding was the result of overprotection compensating for fundamental rejection on the mother's part. As well as compensating for the lack of other satisfactions, eating may also be a method of seeking to gain the mother's approval. Bruch realised later (1957) that these 40 children chosen by their willingness to co-operate demonstrated a neurotic motive and this therefore increased the incidence of neurosis in the sample.

This study of poor children in a large American city a generation ago will not bear direct comparison with the suburban English children in the author's practice, but the basic picture of children from unhappy homes obtaining some satisfaction from eating is true of both groups.

The high proportion of only children or youngest was probably a factor peculiar to a part of New York at this time, as Johnson, Burke & Mayer (1956) found no significant difference in family placing and number of siblings between 28 obese high school girls and 28 normal controls in 1956, and less than half of the author's series were only children or youngest.

Although the author's main series is a small one of 19 children aged eight to 19, consisting of 14 girls and five boys, the children and adolescents are all well known to him and in most cases there is an obvious psychological cause for compensatory over-eating. Seven of the children come from broken homes and one is a foster child. Three have only one parent living, but two of these are happy. Of the remaining nine children four have obviously unhappy relationships with one or both parents, and another put on weight at the onset of epilepsy. These 19 obese children have been compared with controls matched for age and sex. Only one of the controls comes from a broken home, one is a foster child and five others appeared to the author to be unhappy. Thus 14 of the obese children appeared to be obviously unhappy compared with seven of the controls, only one of whom is obese.

Bullen, Read & Mayer (1964) found that 18 per cent of their 109 obese high school girls came from homes with one parent missing, compared with 4 per cent of the non-obese controls.

Obesity commencing at puberty in girls may be associated with a psychological rejection of the idea of pregnancy, according to Hilde Bruch. Increasing emotional maturity can cause a girl to ' grow out of ' this type of obesity (see Cases 6 and 7 on page 168; Case 2 possibly comes into this category, as the pregnancy was unplanned).

THE PROGNOSIS OF CHILDHOOD OBESITY

Transient obesity. Many babies pass through a phase of fatness before they become physically active and start to lose weight by crawling and walking. In some boy babies the mother is worried because the penis is hidden behind the fat on the mons pubis, and unmasking it by pressure on the mons will relieve her anxiety. In most fat babies, unless they are being deliberately overfed by a parent, no treatment is needed beyond ensuring an adequate protein intake and a minimum of sugar and products containing it.

Some pre-adolescent children, especially boys, develop moderate obesity which they lose during the growth spurt at 13 to 15 years of age in boys, and 11 to 13 years of age in girls.

Long-term prognosis. It has been stated that four-fifths of overweight children will become obese adults, but this statement is based on the findings of Haase & Hoseneld (1956) quoted by Lloyd *et al.* (1961) that four-fifths of 50 patients followed up from an original sample of 335 were obese, i.e. only 14 per cent were followed up and no really valid conclusions can be drawn from this. Abraham & Nordsieck (1960) whose results have been widely quoted in American literature followed up 100 overweight children and 100 normal children aged 10 to 13 years and located 174 of them 20 years later. They used 120 of these in their survey and added replacements to bring them up to their original numbers. Their findings were that:

    43 out of 50 obese boys became obese adults.

    21 out of 50 average weight boys became obese adults.

    40 out of 50 obese girls became obese adults.

    9 out of 50 average weight girls became obese adults.

Lloyd and her colleagues in Birmingham (1961) followed up nine years later 67 of 98 children who had attended an overweight clinic at a children's hospital in 1950. Over half of the boys, then aged 18 years were still overweight, and about three-quarters of the girls, then aged $17\frac{1}{2}$, were still overweight, so that about two-thirds of the total series were likely to become obese adults. The whole group had been treated intensively with diet and amphetamine sulphate for about a year, but very few had attended thereafter. An interesting finding is that at the final examination the mean-overweight of the patients whose weight after intensive treatment had returned to near normal, did not differ significantly from that of the children whose weight had responded less satisfactorily to the treatment. In other words intensive treatment for a year had had no appreciable effect on the prognosis when fully grown.

Asher (1966) found that of 28 children obese at five years of age 16 were still obese at the age of 10. Lorber (1966) followed up 53 of his 68 extremely obese children aged three to 15 for one to three and a half years; only seven were much improved or normal, 23 others were improved but still very obese and 23 were still extremely obese.

Of the author's small group of 19 children, 13 have been followed up for five to 10 years, and six for three or four years only. They show a total of 12 successes, four relapses, and three failures. Most of the successful youngsters managed on diet alone, and they included four out of five boys. Only in five of the successes can treatment have made a positive contribution to success (Cases 2, 6, 10, 15, 17), and in the remainder the lessening of a stressful situation was likely to be the most important factor for success. Eight of the 11 successes in the author's series occurred in their late teens (Cases 2, 6, 7, 10, 12, 15, 17, 19) so that the prognosis may not be so bad as suggested by Lloyd's series which is the only long-term British follow-up.

Case histories

Classification of the result in each case is based on the same criteria as in the main series (p. 120) using the weight charts specially prepared for Tanner *et al* (1966) by Creaseys of Hertford as the standard for normality.

1. Andrea, aged 17, was working full time and keeping house for her father and younger brother, who were not easy to get on with. Her mother had left home. Andrea was 95 kg. (209 lb.) and lost 6·4 kg. (14 lb.) in eight weeks on diet alone and a further 7·7 kg. (17 lb.) in another 13 weeks with Dexten. Six months later she had regained half the loss, and three years later had regained all but 4·1 kg. (9 lb.) of the original 14 kg. (31 lb.) lost. *Relapsed success.*

2. Brenda—Andrea's older sister, aged 19, was living with the embittered separated mother and her man friend whom Brenda disliked. She weighed 75·5 kg. (167 lb.), of which she lost 4·5 kg. (10 lb.) after ten weeks on a diet; after 3½ years she was 68 kg. (151 lb.). *Success.*

3. Charles, aged 10, was pampered by his semi-invalid mother and his maternal grandmother who constantly clashed with his father, a tense person who was often depressed. His sister was a typical mixed-up teenager. Charles' 49 kg. (108 lb.) increased by 5·9 kg. (13 lb.) in seven months while on a diet, but seven years later when his sister had left home, he had grown out of his obesity and was within normal limits at 81 kg. (178 lb.). *Success.*

4. Diana, aged 14, who weighed 84 kg. (186 lb.), lost 10·5 kg. (23 lb.) in 12 weeks on a diet and a further 1·8 kg. (4 lb.) in another four weeks. Four years later she was 86 kg. (190 lb.). *Partial success and relapse.*

5. Elizabeth, aged 18, was 81·5 kg. (180 lb.) and lost 3·6 kg. (8 lb.) in five weeks on diet. Two years later she was 83·5 kg. (184 lb.) and lost 3·2 kg. (7 lb.) with a diet. Three years later she was 72 kg. (159 lb.). *Success.*

6. Frances, aged 14, was living with her mother and maternal grandparents, as her father, to whom she was very attached, had left home. Her grandparents preferred her older sister to her, and eating sweets helped to compensate. Of her 79·5 kg. (176 lb.) she lost only 0·5 kg. (1 lb.) in two weeks by dieting, but another 5 kg. (11 lb.) in eight weeks with the aid of phenmetrazine. A year later she was 90 kg. (198 lb.) but two years later she was 102 kg. (225·5 lb.). She has now dieted with complete success losing 38 kg. (83·5 lb.) in 60 weeks to be within 10 per cent of her ' best ' weight. *Success.* (p. 69.)

7. Gail, aged 16, lived with her mother and step-father who was an unstable individual. The mother had no real control over Gail. She was 65 kg. (144 lb.), lost no weight on diet, but with chlorphentermine lost 4·1 kg. (9 lb.) in four weeks. She had maintained 3·2 kg. (7 lb.) of weight loss 18 months later but after two years was only 53 kg. (117 lb.), explaining that she had taken her dieting seriously because she had a regular boy friend. *Success.*

8. Harold, aged 8 and weighing 40 kg. (88 lb.), had a sister 12 months old and did not get on well with his father. At 10 he was 49 kg. (108 lb.) and at 11, 55 kg. (121 lb.), but at 13 years of age he was 63 kg. (139 lb.) and within normal limits for his height and age. *Success.*

9. Irene, aged 13, was 78·5 kg. (173 lb.) and lost 5·9 kg. (13 lb.)

in 13 weeks. At 17 she was 86 kg. (190 lb.). *Partial success and relapse.*

10. Jennifer, aged 15, was the third of four children brought up very happily by their widowed mother. She lost 11·3 kg. (25 lb.) of her 85 kg. (188 lb.) in 21 weeks; 3½ years later she was 69·5 kg. (153 lb.) and at 20 she was still only 75 kg. (166 lb.). *Success.*

11. Karen, aged 9, lived mainly with her maternal grand-parents but occasionally with her mother and a man friend, who eventually became her step-father. Karen was 47 kg. (104 lb.) at 9, 48·5 kg. (107 lb.) at 10, 54 kg. (120 lb.) at 15. *Success.*

12. Leslie, aged 16, was a foster child who gave his foster-parents a lot of trouble. His weight of 100 kg. (220 lb.) went down to 87 kg. (192 lb.) in six months, and to 81 kg. (178 lb.) in a year. He maintained this weight for three further years. *Success.*

13. Maurice, aged 11, had a domineering mother and an unassertive father. Maurice came under the care of the Child Guidance Clinic because of persistent school refusal. He was 53·5 kg. (118 lb.) and dieting with his mother, who was one of the successes in the main series he lost 4·5 kg. (10 lb.) in 10 weeks and had maintained this weight loss 12 months later. After two years he was 60 kg. (133 lb.) and after another five years he was 79·5 kg. (176 lb.). *Partial success and relapse.*

14. Naomi, aged 17, weighing 65 kg. (143 lb.) lost 2·7 kg. (6 lb.) in four days initially. After 3½ years she was 70 kg. 154 lb.). Her father was dead but she was happy with her mother. *Failure.*

15. Olive, aged 19, lost 4·5 kg. (10 lb.) of her 68·8 kg. (152 lb.) only with the aid of amphetamine, but had maintained this weight loss six months later, and was the same weight three years later. She had an unhappy relationship with her mother who suffered from chronic anxiety and depression. *Partial success.*

16. Patricia, aged 10, was living with her mother and brother, the father having deserted the family. She was 53 kg. (117 lb.) and had been obese since the age of six when her father left them. Three years later she was 70 kg. (154 lb.) but after another two years she was a happy 15-year-old and weighed only 65 kg. (143 lb.). *Success.*

17. Rhoda, 18, was living with her grandparents as her mother and father had separated. She was 71 kg. (157 lb.). Six months later she was 71·5 kg. (158 lb.) but four years later was 67·5 kg. (149 lb.) *Success*.

18. Sally, aged 19, lived with her widowed mother and invalid grandmother. She had been 94 kg. (207 lb.) at the age of 14 and was now 79 kg. (174 lb.). In spite of dieting and phenmetrazine intermittently she was 85 kg. (187 lb.) after two years. *Failure*.

19. Trevor was 11 when he developed epilepsy incompletely controlled by drugs. He began to put on weight soon after this and when 13 was put on a diet. This was ineffective, but with the aid of phenmetrazine he lost 5 kg. (11 lb.) in 13 weeks; he regained 5·4 kg. (12 lb.) in the next five months. He was growing fast and had no epileptic attacks in the succeeding four months during which he lost 0·9 kg. (2 lb.) without drugs. *Partial success*.

As many as six of the 19 children failed to lose weight when put on a diet initially, showing the initial lack of motivation, as only one out of every nine adults failed.

TREATMENT

Hilde Bruch emphasises that treatment can only be successful if a child wants to lose weight. Whereas most obese adults present themselves because they want to lose weight, most children are brought by a parent without necessarily having any personal desire to lose weight. Of eight teenagers who came to the author themselves, six were successful after three to 10 years, while of five who were brought by their parents only one was successful. Eating or not eating is one of the common ways in which children defy their parents, and it is essential to try and convince parents that they should display great tact over a fat child's appetite. To attempt to pressurise a child into cutting down his food intake when eating is his main pleasure in life, is unkind and may be harmful. If he already feels rejected and guilty this feeling may be intensified especially if there is any ' disturbance of the body image ' (p. 104). It is therefore especially important in children to make a full assessment of the situation and gain the child's co-operation.

A full history should be taken modifying the questionnaire on page 111 to suit each individual child, and asking the child questions as well as the parent. Feeding habits and parental attitudes to food intake should be elucidated. A brief medical examination does not need to include the estimation of blood pressure or the testing of the urine. The height and weight can be plotted on a growth chart.

As with adults, many obese children eat no more than their peers. Exercise is therefore important, but it is often difficult for a fat child to exercise more, as he is often teased by his companions about his weight, appearance and slowness of movement and this may discourage him from taking part in group play. Swimming is perhaps the most useful form of exercise for a fat child to take, and walking can be encouraged by the parents, but extra exercise should be taken daily to be of benefit (Chap. 8).

Diet

A free form of diet is essential for children and it is important that the whole family should attempt to alter its eating habits to conform with the child's needs if success is to be obtained. Whilst growth is in progress it may indeed be dangerous to subject children or adolescents to long term low calorie diets. Wolff (1955) showed that during rapid weight reduction, obese children gained less height than was expected.

Drugs

These are commonly indicated if a pre-adolescent or adolescent child has a genuine desire to lose weight. All the major anorectic drugs are effective in 80 to 90 per cent of cases and side-effects are minimal.

Amphetamine resinate did not cause restlessness or excitability in a dose of 12·5 mg. daily in any of the 68 children in Lorber's trial; 61 lost an average of 1·9 kg. (4·2 lb.) in a month.

Phenmetrazine was used in 21 children receiving an unrestricted diet; 18 lost weight while only two lost on the placebo. The dose was half a tablet b.d. under eight years of age and 1 b.d. over eight years of age (Rendall-Short, 1960). Of 51 children, 39 had lost weight after two months in Fischman's trial (1965) and in Lorber's series 52 out of 61 lost an average of 1 kg. (2·2 lb.) in a month.

Diethylpropion 2 tablets daily caused an average loss of weight of 2·25 kg. (5 lb.) in two months in 28 out of 33 children (Everley Jones, 1962). Andelmann *et al* (1967) found that 37 out of 51 adolescents who wanted to lose weight lost more than 0·45 kg. (1 lb.) per week for 11 weeks. No side-effects occurred which were not also caused by the placebo.

Phentermine was the most successful of the drugs used in Lorber's 68 obese children, as it caused weight loss averaging 1·3 kg. (2·9 lb.) per month in no less than 64 of them.

Fenfluramine is probably the least likely of all the major drugs to lead to habit formation, and it may well become the drug of choice in children, especially if its effect on metabolism is confirmed.

Group therapy

This is particularly applicable to children, as most of them depend to a large extent on the approval of their associates. As the treatment of childhood obesity had only yielded a 10 per cent success rate in the New York City Health Department's Bureau of Nutrition, a controlled trial of group treatment was undertaken at a Junior High School in Brooklyn (Christakis, 1967). Of 90 obese 13/14-year-old boys, 55 were randomly selected as the experimental group and 35 as the control group. The experimental group had twice-weekly talks on diet and nutrition after school hours and special exercises during school hours in addition to the usual school physical training programme. After the end of 18 months those boys who were more than 30 per cent overweight in the experimental group had gained an average of 2·6 kg. (5·8 lb.) while those in the control group had gained an average of 6·1 kg. (13·5 lb.). This represented an 11 per cent decrease in the average degree of overweight in the experimental group compared with a 2 per cent decrease in the controls.

Four groups for girls between 10 and 16 years of age were formed in 1965 by the Public Health Department of Croydon and met fortnightly with a woman doctor. Of the first 59 girls nine attained their ideal weight and 28 others lost weight

while six left the area or started work, and one was discovered
to be a diabetic: approximately two-thirds therefore responded
satisfactorily to treatment (Mortimer, 1968).

REFERENCES

ABRAHAMS, A. & NORDSIECK, M. (1960). Relationship of excess weight in
children and adults. *Publ. Hlth Rep.* **75,** 263.
ANDELMAN, M. B., JONES, C. & NATHAN, S. (1967). Treatment of obesity in
under privileged adolescents. Comparison of diethylpropion hydrochloride with placebo. *Clin. Pediat.* **6,** 327.
ASHER, P. (1966). Fat babies and fat children. The prognosis of obesity in
the very young. *Archs Dis. Childh.* **41,** 672.
BRUCH, H. (1957). *The Importance of Overweight.* New York: Norton.
BRUCH, H. & TORRAINE, G. (1960). Obesity in childhood. V. The family frame
of obese children. *Psychosom. Med.* **2,** 141.
BULLEN, B. A., REED, R. B. & MAYER, J. (1964). Physical activity of obese
and non-obese adolescent girls appraised by motion picture sampling.
Am. J. clin. Nutr. **14,** 211.
CHRISTAKIS, G. (1967). Community programs for weight reduction: Experi-
ence of the Bureau of Nutrition, New York City. *Can. J. Publ. Hlth,* **58,**
499.
ELLIS, R. W. B., & TALLERMAN, K. H. (1934). Obesity in childhood. *Lancet,*
2, 615.
FISCHMAN, M. E. (1965). Control of obesity in children. *J. med. Soc. New Jers.*
62, 18.
GRANT, M. W. (1966). Juvenile obesity—chronic, progressive and transient.
Med. Off. **153,** 331.
JAMES, G. & CHRISTAKIS, G. (1966). New York City Bureau of Nutrition
current programs and research activities. *J. Am. Diet. Ass.* **48,** 301.
JOHNSON, M. L., BURKE, B. S. & MAYER, J. (1956). Relative importance of
inactivity and overeating in the energy balance of obese high school
girls. *Am. J. clin. Nutr.* **4,** 37.
JONES, H. EVERLEY, (1962). A trial of diethylpropion in the treatment of
childhood obesity. *Practitioner,* **188,** 229.
LLOYD, J. K., WOLFF, O. H. & WHELAN, W. S. (1961). Childhood obesity. A
long term study of height and weight. *Br. med. J.* **2,** 145.
LORBER, J. (1966). A controlled trial of anorectic drugs. *Archs Dis. childh.*
41, 309.
MORTIMER, P. M. (1968). An approach to the treatment of the obese school-
child. *Proc. Nutr. Soc.* **27,** 29.
RENDLE-SHORT, J. (1960). Obesity in childhood. A clinical trial of phenmetrazine. *Br. med. J.* **1,** 703.
TANNER, J. M., WHITEHOUSE, R. H. & TAKAISHI, M. (1966). Standards from
birth to maturity for height, weight, height velocity and weight velocity.
British children, 1965. *Archs Dis. Childh.* **41,** 454, 613.
WOLFF, O. H. (1955). Obesity in childhood; study of birth weight, height
and onset of puberty. *Q. Jl Med.* **24,** 109.

CHAPTER 16

The Obese Diabetic

DIABETICS are usually placed in one of two main groups, the characteristics of which are summarised below.

Group I. Juvenile diabetes. This type of diabetes is probably due to an absolute or almost absolute lack of insulin. It presents acutely in children and young adults with the classical symptomatology of thirst, polyuria and loss of weight.

Group II. Maturity onset diabetes. This type of diabetes, due to a relative lack of insulin or an insensitivity to insulin, presents gradually in older adults who are usually obese. In many cases there are no symptoms, the diagnosis being made on routine urine testing. Individuals presenting in this manner who are not obese, form a small sub-group. Recent research appears to indicate that these individuals should perhaps be classed as members of group I, with a late onset of symptoms, as their metabolism is different from that of the obese members of group II.

Elevated serum insulin levels following oral glucose did not occur in non-obese patients with maturity onset diabetes, or in obese patients with maturity onset diabetes who had reduced their weight to normal (Karam *et al.*, 1965). They only occurred in 4 out of 24 non-obese normal patients with a strong family history of diabetes (Grodsky *et al.*, 1965). This appears to show that elevated serum insulin levels are associated with obesity rather than with the diabetic state, as it has been stated previously that most obese diabetics have raised serum insulin levels even when fasting (p. 39). As outlined previously therefore, obesity appears to lead to insulin resistance which after many years brings about the diabetic state (group II type) in subjects with an hereditary tendency.

Medley, among others, suggests on the contrary, that the diabetic tendency manifests itself first as obesity, and in support cites his findings (Medley, 1965) that young women with a family history of diabetes and/or who had produced babies over 4 kg. (9 lb.) in weight all showed gross impairment of glucose tolerance after prednisolone whereas only about one half of obese patients with a similar history showed this impairment. It does not seem justifiable, however, to compare the young women, who may eventually proceed to group I type diabetes, with the obese patients who may become group II type diabetics. Moreover the sociological and statistical evidence suggesting that obesity causes diabetes is massive.

Obesity as an aetiological factor in maturity onset diabetes

Long continued obesity with its high intake of carbohydrates, especially sucrose, leads almost invariably to an abnormal glucose tolerance test with a raised blood glucose level; after 18 years all of Ogilvie's 11 cases showed this (Ogilvie, 1935). In a proportion of individuals obesity leads to frank diabetes (three of Ogilvie's cases). Three of the author's obese patients, women who had been obese for 24 years, 27 years and over 30 years respectively, became diabetic during the course of a $7\frac{1}{2}$-10 year follow-up. In two of them rapid weight loss occurred without a change of dietary habit, and in the third a persistent monilial infection of the vagina was the presenting symptom; she still has a weight problem. Two other patients with long standing obesity who had not sought treatment for their overweight developed diabetes during the same period.

Joslin et al. (1959) found that 77 per cent of 1,000 consecutive diabetics were obese. From 1898 to 1928 among 4,596 patients aged 20 years and over, 78·5 per cent of the males and 83·3 per cent of the females were at one time overweight prior to the onset of their diabetes and no less than 16·5 per cent of the men and 25·8 per cent of the women were 40 per cent or more overweight by the Metropolitan Life Insurance Company's standards. In maturity onset diabetes, i.e. diabetes in persons of 40 years of age and over, obesity is almost invariably a precursor. Only two patients out of 252 whose onset was in the fifties were below standard weight in Joslin's series and 87 per cent were above standard weight. In 24 cases of conjugal diabetes only one of the 27 partners seen by Joslin himself was thin, and he concluded that ' they contracted the disease from exposure to good food rather than to one another.' The greater frequency of diabetes in city workers in contradistinction to country workers can be explained by obesity.

Yudkin (1964) states that there is a time lag of approximately 20 years between a dietary cause and the onset of diabetes, which is in keeping with Ogilvie's evidence. Yudkin showed that in many different countries there was a highly significant association between the intake of sugar before 1939 and the incidence of diabetes, as shown by Joslin's figures, in 1955 to 1956. Cleave & Campbell (1966) also give evidence to show a correlation between a high intake of sugar and diabetes in many different countries, and see also Cohen's evidence (p. 37). Yudkin found a small but insignificant correlation between pre-war fat intake and later diabetes.

Diabetes is rare in eskimos who take no sugar and live almost entirely on fat meat (Jackson, 1964).

Treatment of the obese diabetic

Diabetics have a strong incentive to lose weight and keep fit. In addition to reducing the incidence of complications and ensuring a longer span of life, weight reduction may also save them from daily insulin injections. Nevertheless diabetics are subject to the same social pressures as are other obese people, and many of them have the same need to eat in compensation for something lacking in their personal life. The same routine for assessment of their problem of overweight should therefore be followed as for other obese people (Chap. 10) and treatment can include the use of drugs if necessary. Fineberg (1961) found phenmetrazine to be unquestionably superior to diethylpropion in a controlled cross over trial on 42 obese diabetics over a period of 12 weeks; the weight loss with phenmetrazine was more than double that with diethylpropion.

In patients who have real difficulty in maintaining weight loss there remain the weight reducing oral hypoglycaemic agents phenformin and metformin (pp. 82 & 84) but a vigorous attempt should be made to initiate and maintain weight loss by routine measures before these are used.

REFERENCES

CLEAVE, T. L. & CAMPBELL, G. D. (1966). *Diabetes, Coronary Thrombosis and the Saccharine Disease*. Bristol: Wright.

FINEBERG, S. K. (1961). Obesity, diabetes and anorexigenics. *J. Am. med. Ass.* **175**, 680.

GRODSKY, G. M., KARAM, J. H. & PAVLATOS, F. C. (1965). Serum insulin response to glucose in pre-diabetic subjects. *Lancet*, **1**, 290.

JACKSON, W. P. U. (1964). *On Diabetes Mellitus*. Springfield, Illinois: Thomas.

JOSLIN, E. P., ROOT, H. F., WHITE, P. & MARBLE, A. (1959). *The treatment of Diabetes Mellitus*. 16th Ed. London: Kimpton.

KARAM, J. H., GRODSKY, G. M. & PAVLATOS, F. C. (1965). Critical factors in excessive seru-insulin response to glucose in obesity and maturity onset diabetes. *Lancet*, **1**, 286.

MEDLEY, D. R. K. (1965). The relationship between diabetes and obesity. *Q. Jl Med.* **34**, 111.

OGILVIE, R. F. (1935). Sugar tolerance in obese subjects. A review of 65 cases. *Q. Jl Med.* **28**, 345.

YUDKIN, J. (1964). Dietary fat and dietary sugar in relation to ischaemic heart disease and diabetes. *Lancet*, **2**, 4.

CHAPTER 17

The Future

PRESENT-DAY methods of tackling the vast problems of obesity in the Western world are merely scratching the surface of the problem. In Great Britain the sugar consumption per head per annum rose from 14 lb. in 1815 to 120 lb. in 1965. An enlightened government could reduce the national intake of sugar by cutting down imports and controlling advertising by the major media. It could bring strong pressure to bear on the community to take more regular exercise and it could encourage local authorities to increase the number of obesity clinics. This type of government, however, is unlikely to emerge during the present generation in any of the major countries, and the control of obesity is likely to rest mainly with individual physicians. Apart from attempting to help individual patients with weight problems on the lines outlined previously, there seem to be three aspects of patient care which afford some prospects of major improvement.

Ante-natal weight control

If special attention is focused on the weight of all pregnant women during the middle trimester when at least half of them are likely to need dietetic advice, the young families of the future will be more likely to realise the dangers of a high carbohydrate, and especially a high sucrose, intake.

The control of childhood obesity

There are ample opportunities in family and hospital practice for physicians with the care of small children to give dietary advice to those parents whose babies and children appear to be developing clinical obesity. The present tendency is to increase the carbohydrate intake of babies at the expense of protein and fat by replacing milk with high carbohydrate cereal often before three months of age. Pressure should be brought to bear to reverse this tendency.

Parents should be advised for various reasons to reduce the present high intake of sugar in the form of sweets, ice cream and cake.

If children are eating to compensate for lack of affection the physician can endeavour to modify the parents' attitudes, enlisting the help of Child Guidance staff or psychiatrists if necessary.

Group therapy

The problem of the middle aged obese woman might come nearer solution if each family doctor or hospital physician would set up one or more groups of six to 10 women meeting weekly under a leader appointed by themselves, in a place where there are social facilities as well as contact with nursing and/or medical staff.

The Obesity Association

In this country the recently formed Obesity Association, which has the backing of many of the leading experts in the field of research into the aetiology and treatment of obesity, as well as several Members of Parliament may be welded into a body which can have a major influence on the future of the obese population in this country.

Appendix I

STATISTICAL BULLETIN METROPOLITAN LIFE INSURANCE COMPANY NO. 40
NOVEMBER - DECEMBER, 1959
DESIRABLE WEIGHTS IN INDOOR CLOTHING

MEN AGED 25 AND OVER

Height	Weight (lb.)		
	Small frame	Medium frame	Large frame
5′ 2″	112-120	118-129	126-141
3″	115-123	121-133	129-144
4″	118-126	124-136	132-148
5″	121-129	127-139	135-152
6″	124-133	130-143	138-156
7″	128-137	134-147	142-161
8″	132-141	138-152	147-166
9″	136-145	142-156	151-169
10″	140-150	146-160	155-174
11″	144-154	150-165	159-179
6′ 0″	148-158	154-170	164-184
1″	152-162	156-175	168-189
2″	156-167	162-180	173-194
3″	160-171	167-185	178-199
4″	164-175	172-190	182-204

WOMEN AGED 25 AND OVER

Height	Weight (lb.)		
	Small frame	Medium frame	Large frame
4′ 10″	92- 98	96-107	104-119
11″	94-101	98-110	106-122
5′ 0″	96-104	101-113	109-125
1″	99-107	104-116	112-128
2″	102-110	107-119	115-131
3″	105-113	110-122	118-134
4″	108-116	113-126	121-138
5″	111-119	116-130	125-142
6″	114-123	120-135	129-146
7″	118-127	124-139	133-150
8″	122-131	128-143	137-154
9″	126-135	132-147	141-158
10″	130-140	136-151	145-163
11″	134-144	140-155	149-168
6′ 0″	139-148	144-159	153-173

DESIRABLE WEIGHT (METRIC SYSTEM) IN INDOOR CLOTHING

MEN AGED 25 AND OVER

| Height | Weight (kg.) | | |
	Small frame	Medium frame	Large frame
5′ 2″	50·5-54·5	53·5-58·5	57·0-64·0
3″	52·0-56·0	55·0-61·0	58·5-65·0
4″	53·5-57·0	56·0-62·0	60·0-67·0
5″	55·0-58·5	57·5-63·0	61·0-69·0
6″	56·0-60·0	58·5-65·0	62·5-71·0
7″	58·0-62·0	56·0-66·5	64·5-73·0
8″	60·0-64·0	62·5-69·0	66·5-75·0
9″	62·0-66·0	64·5-71·0	68·5-77·0
10″	63·5-68·0	66·0-72·5	70·0-79·0
11″	65·0-70·0	68·0-75·0	72·0-81·0
6′ 0″	67·0-71·5	70·0-77·0	74·0-83·5
1″	69·0-73·5	71·5-79·0	76·0-85·5
2″	71·0-76·0	73·5-81·5	78·5-88·0
3″	72·5-77·5	76·0-79·0	80·5-90·5
4″	74·0-79·0	78·0-86·0	82·5-92·5

WOMEN AGED 25 AND OVER

| Height | Weight (kg.) | | |
	Small frame	Medium frame	Large frame
4′ 10″	42·0-44·5	43·5-48·5	47·0-54·0
11″	42·5-46·0	44·5-50·0	48·0-55·0
5′ 0″	43·5-47·0	46·0-51·0	49·5-56·5
1″	45·0-48·5	47·0-52·5	51·0-58·0
2″	46·5-50·0	48·5-54·0	52·0-59·5
3″	47·5-51·0	50·0-55·0	53·5-61·0
4″	49·0-52·5	51·0-57·0	55·0-62·0
5″	50·5-54·0	52·5-58·5	57·0-64·5
6″	52·0-56·0	54·5-61·0	58·5-66·0
7″	53·5-57·5	56·0-63·0	60·0-68·0
8″	55·0-59·5	58·0-65·0	62·0-70·0
9″	57·0-61·0	60·0-66·5	64·0-71·5
10″	58·5-63·5	62·0-68·5	66·0-74·0
11″	61·0-65·0	63·5-70·0	67·5-76·0
6′ 0″	63·0-67·0	65·0-72·0	69·5-78·5

Appendix II

CALORIE VALUE OF COMMON FOODSTUFFS

Taken from *The Composition of Foods* Medical Research Council's Special Report No. 297 by R. A. McCance and E. W. Widdowson (Second Impression 1967). All values are for foods as eaten unless otherwise shown. Cooked fruit should be stewed without added sugar, and may be sweetened with saccharine. Each carbohydrate unit is the approximate equivalent of 5 gm. of carbohydrate.

Product	Calories per oz.	Average portion	Calories per portion	Carbo-hydrate units
FRUIT				
Apples	13	one	60	2
Apricots, fresh	8	4 oz.	32	0
stewed without sugar	6	4 oz.	24	1
canned, sweetened	30	4 oz.	120	5
dried, raw	52	2 oz.	104	2·5
cooked without sugar	17	4 oz.	68	0
Avocados	25	½ (3 oz.)	75	1
Bananas	22	1 (4 oz.)	88	5
Blackberries, fresh	8	4 oz.	32	2
Cherries, fresh	11	4 oz.	44	3
Cranberry Sauce	60	1 oz.	60	2·5
Dates, dried	70			4
Figs, dried raw, stewed without sugar	30			3
Fruit cocktail, canned in syrup	27	4 oz.	108	6
Gooseberries, fresh ripe	10	4 oz.	40	2
Grapes, fresh	17	3 oz.	51	3
Grapefruit, fresh (whole fruit)	3	½ (4 oz.)	12	1
Lemon juice	2			
Loganberries, stewed without sugar	4	4 oz.	16	1
Melons	4-7	6 oz.	24-42	2
Olives, green, in brine	24	4 (1 oz.)	24	0
Oranges, fresh	10	1 (6 oz.)	60	3
Orange juice	11	4 oz.	44	2
Peaches, fresh	11	1 (4 oz.)	44	2
canned, sweetened	25	4 oz.	100	4

182

Product	Calories per oz.	Average portion	Calories per portion	Carbo-hydrate units
Pears, fresh	9	1 (5 oz.)	45	2·5
canned, sweetened	22	4 oz.	88	4
Pineapple, fresh	13	4 oz.	52	2
canned, sweetened	22	4 oz.	88	5
Plums, fresh	10	2 oz.	20	1
canned, sweetened	22	4 oz.	88	4
Prunes, stewed without sugar	19	4 oz.	76	4
Raisins, dried	70	1 oz.	70	4
Raspberries, fresh or stewed without sugar	7	4 oz.	28	4
Rhubarb, fresh raw	2	4 oz.	8	0
Strawberries, fresh	7	4 oz.	28	1·5
Sultanas	71	1 oz.	71	2
VEGETABLES				
Asparagus, fresh	5	4 oz. (8 spears)	20	0·5
canned	3	4 oz.	12	0·5
Beans, baked	26	4 oz.	104	4
broad	12	4 oz.	48	3
french or runner	2	4 oz.	8	0·5
haricot, boiled	25	4 oz.	100	4
Beetroot, boiled	13	2 oz.	26	1
Broccoli, fresh	4	4 oz.	16	0
Brussels sprouts, fresh boiled	5	3 oz.	15	0
Cabbage, fresh boiled	2	4 oz.	8	0
Carrots, fresh	6	3 oz.	18	1
canned	5	3 oz.	15	1
Cauliflower, fresh boiled	3	4 oz.	12	0·5
Celery, stalk raw	3	3 oz.	9	0
Chicory and endives	3	3 oz.	9	0
Corn, Sweet, fresh boiled	24	4 oz.	96	4
Cucumbers, fresh	3	2 oz.	6	0
Leeks, leaves	7	4 oz.	28	1
Lentils, dried	104	1½ oz.	104	3
Lettuce	3	¼ oz.	1	0
Marrow	2	6 oz.	12	0
Mushrooms	2	2 oz.	4	0
Onions, fresh boiled	4	4 oz.	16	0·5
fried	101	2 oz.	202	1
Parsnips, fresh	16	4 oz.	64	2
Peas, fresh	14	4 oz.	56	2
Potatoes, chips	68	4 oz.	272	4
boiled	23	4 oz.	92	4
crisps	159	1 oz.	159	1
roast	35	4 oz.	140	4

Product	Calories per oz.	Average portion	Calories per portion	Carbo- hydrate units
Radishes, fresh	4	2 oz.	8	0
Spinach, fresh or canned	7	4 oz.	28	0
Tomatoes, fresh	4	4 oz.	16	0·5
Tomato sauce or ketchup	28	1 oz.	28	1
Turnips, fresh and greens	3	3 oz.	9	1
Watercress	4	1 oz.	4	0
NUTS				
Various, dried	156-189	1 oz.	156-189	1
Chestnuts, fresh	49	2 oz.	96	4
CEREALS and their products				
Barley	102	1 oz.	102	4
Biscuits, plain	123	2 oz.	226	8
sweet	158	2 oz.	316	7
Bread	65-72	1 slice	65-72	3
Cake, fruit	110/141	2 oz.	220/282	6
Cornflakes, Rice Crispies Shredded Wheat, Weetabix	100/104	1 oz.	100/104	5
Cornflour	100	1 oz.	100	5
Energen rolls, Figgerolls	110	2	36	1
Flour, raw	100	1 oz.	100	4
Macaroni, boiled	32	1 oz.	32	5
Milk puddings, various	36/42	8 oz.	320	8
Oatmeal, raw	115	1 oz.	115	4
Pastry, shortcrust	132/157	2 oz.	280	3
Rice, polished raw	102	1 oz.	102	4
Ryvita	34 (per piece)	2 pieces	68	3
Suet pudding	105	6 oz.	630	15
Trifle	43	6 oz.	258	8
Yorkshire pudding	63	4 oz.	252	6
CONFECTIONERY				
Chocolate, milk	167	2 oz.	334	5
plain	155	2 oz.	310	5
Fruit gums	49			2·5
Golden syrup	84	½ oz.	42	2·5
Honey	82			5
Ice Cream	56	2 oz.	112	3
Jams	75	½ oz.	38	2
Jellies, as eaten	23	6 oz.	132	6
Peppermints	111			6
Sugar	112	½ oz.	56	3
Sweets, boiled	93	1 oz.	93	4
Toffees	123			4

Product	Calories per oz.	Average portion	Calories per portion	Carbo-hydrate units
FATS				
Butter	226	¼ oz. (per slice)	55	0
Lard	262	¼ oz.	65	0
Mayonnaise	206	½ oz.	103	0
Peanut Butter	170	¼ oz. (per slice)	43	0
DAIRY PRODUCTS				
Cheese, Camembert	88	1½ oz.	132	0
Cheddar	120	1½ oz.	180	0
Cottage	30	1½ oz.	45	0
Cream	232	1½ oz.	348	0
Cream, single	62	1 oz.	62	0
double	131	1 oz.	131	0
Eggs, whole	46	1 (2 oz.)	92	0
white	13			0
yolk	100			0
fried	68	1 (2 oz.)	136	0
Milk, pasteurised	19	6 oz. (1 cup)	114	1·5
evaporated	45	1 oz.	41	0·5
condensed, sweetened	100	½ oz.	50	2
dried, skimmed	93	6oz. (reconstituted)	60	2
Yoghurt (plain), low fat	15	5 oz.	75	2
MEAT				
Bacon	174	2 oz.	360	0
gammon	92	2 oz.	252	0
Beef, sirloin, roast	109	2 oz.	218	0
Hamburger, fried	104	3 oz.	312	0
stewed steak	58	3 oz.	164	0
corned	66	3 oz.	198	0
Brain, boiled	30	3 oz.	90	0
Chicken, boiled or roast (joint)	54	4 oz.	216	0
Duck, roast	89	4 oz.	35	0
Goose, roast	53	4 oz.	21	0
Gravy, thin	5	2 oz.	10	0
Ham, boiled, lean	62	2 oz.	124	0
Heart	27	3 oz.	81	0
Kidneys, stewed	45	3 oz.	135	0
Lamb, roast leg	83	3 oz.	249	0
chop, grilled	108	3 oz.	324	0
roast shoulder	100	3 oz.	300	0
Liver (ox), fried	81	4 oz.	342	0

Product	Calories per oz.	Average portion	Calories per portion	Carbo-hydrate units
Mutton, roast	83	3 oz.	249	0
Pork, medium fat leg, roast	90	3 oz.	270	0
cutlets, fried	155	3 oz.	465	0
chops, grilled, lean	92	3 oz.	276	0
Sausages, beef, fried	81	3 oz.	243	3
black	81	2 oz.	162	2
breakfast	82	2 oz.	164	2
pork, fried	93	4 oz.	372	3
Steak and kidney pie	90	6 oz.	540	6
Toad-in-the-hole	82	6 oz.	492	6
Turkey, roast	56	2 oz.	112	0
Veal, roast	66	3 oz.	198	0

SEA FOOD

Product	Calories per oz.	Average portion	Calories per portion	Carbo-hydrate units
Cod, steamed	23	8 oz.	184	0
fried	58	8 oz.	464	0
Crab meat	36	3 oz.	108	0
Eel, stewed	106	3 oz.	318	0
Fish paste	49	$\frac{3}{4}$ oz.	36	0
Haddock, steamed	28	6 oz.	168	0
Herring, in vinegar	54	6 oz.	324	0
Lobster	34	3 oz.	102	0
Mackerel, boiled	39	6 oz.	234	0
Oysters, raw	14	(12) 4 oz.	160	0
Pilchards, canned	54	4 oz.	216	0
Plaice, boiled	14	6 oz.	84	0
Prawns, boiled	30	4 oz.	120	0
Salmon, red, fresh, steamed	57	4 oz.	216	0
canned	39	3 oz.	117	0
Sardines, solids + oils	84	2 oz.	168	0
solids, only	60	2 oz.	120	0
Shrimps, boiled	32	4 oz.	128	0
Sole, steamed	24	4 oz.	96	0

MISCELLANEOUS

Product	Calories per oz.	Average portion	Calories per portion	Carbo-hydrate units
Beverages, orange, lemon, grapefruit squashes, various	36/39	2 oz.	72-78	4
Blancmange	34	6 oz.	210	0
Cocoa powder	128	$\frac{1}{2}$ oz.	64	0
Coffee	1	6 oz.	6	0
Doughnuts	101	(1) 4 oz.	404	12
Horlicks	113	$\frac{1}{2}$ oz.	56	1
Jam Roll	115	3 oz.	345	9
Lucozade	19	6 oz.	114	6

Product	Calories per oz.	Average portion	Calories per portion	Carbo- hydrate units
Mince pie	111	(1) 2 oz.	222	5
Ovaltine powder	109	½ oz.	54	1
Ribena	65	2 oz.	130	7
Sausage roll	142	(1) 2 oz.	284	4
Tea	1	6 oz.	6	0
Trifle	42	3 oz.	126	4
ALCOHOL				
Beer, 1 pint	8-11	1 pt.	160-220	4
Champagne	21	3 oz.	63	0
Ciders	11	10 oz.	110	2
Port	43	2 oz.	86	1
Sherry, dry	33	2 oz.	66	0
sweet	38	2 oz.	76	1
Spirits	63	1 oz.	63	0
Stout	10	10 oz.	100	0
Wines, white	21-26	4 oz.	84-102	0
red	18-20	4 oz.	72-80	0

Index

Italic figures indicate the principal references.

189

Printed by John Milne, The Central Press (Aberdeen) Limited, Aberdeen